Men Going Their Own Way
The Anti-Feminism Survival Guide

CHARLES RIVERS

Copyright © 2019 Charles Rivers

All rights reserved.

ISBN: 9781097628322
ISBN-13: 9781097628322

THE RED PILL

"Remember, all I am offering you is the truth, nothing more."

Lawrence Fishburne
The Matrix

CONTENTS

	Acknowledgments	i
1	Beaver Feminist	3
2	Dachshund Feminist	21
3	Weasel Feminist	35
4	Panther Feminist	60
5	Barracuda Feminist	90
6	Iguana Feminist	102
7	Black Widow Feminist	130
8	Cobra Feminist	144

ACKNOWLEDGMENTS

In this book, I would like to thank all of the many adult men who have lent me their childhood/life stories as an example to others on how the red pill awakening process takes place.

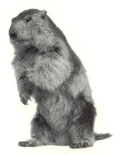

Beaver Feminist
(The *Sex Manipulator*)

*"The illustriously sexy Beaver Feminist uses her
Erotic attractiveness in order to shut down the male thinking processes
so she can fleece him of everything he worked so hard to build."*

Charles Rivers

If you want to regain dominion over a life that is currently being controlled by your dick, then you are going to have to be honest with yourself. You are going to have to be genuine with the belief that you are weaker sexually when in the company of the weaker sex. You will never be able to truly call yourself an MGTOW man if you cannot be a man first. If you are to be what Seinfeld referred to as, *"the Master of Your Domain,"* you must master your entire body and not just your mind. In your current relationships or your pursuit of sex, are you in love with the girl's heart or her big booty? Many men have risked an entire lifetime of happiness for grief. Probably, like you, they were hoping that the girl they chose was not the kind of chick that would destroy their promising dreams.

But if you are taking a bet on a gender that now sees men's hearts as something to rip-apart as opposed to mending together then I know of a casino in Vegas where you could get better odds in gambling.

Simply preparing for the worst in the quest for love and hoping for the best is not a good recipe for entering a relationship in a feminist society. Many of us find out this the hard way that there is no class to weed out which chick really loves us and which one is using us. So it is with this MGTOW manual that I hope to impart with you, what to do if you are in a relationship that is not giving you what you want; or if you are simply seeking to get laid by the opposite gender. Additionally, we will address the final stage of MGTOW for those bro's who have sworn women off their menu list because they are tired of them wrecking the hell out of their lives and finances.

I believe for any of these three journeys you will need advice from someone who is level-headed on this subject and not just espousing anger. The main thing you learn by the time you become a Sergeant in the U.S. Cavalry is that you must be able to think on your feet and in the worst circumstances you can imagine; including combat. I want you to keep this advice in mind as you absorb the tenants of the M.G.T.O.W. Movement. No organization, to include this one has ever stood the test of time with violence or anger as its cornerstone. Test this theory if you must throughout the history of the world from slavery to feminism and you will find an idea that is on the outs with the masses of violence intolerable people.

The last thing the MGTOW Movement wants to come off as is a masculine version of the current Radical Feminist Movement. Let me give you my background outside of the military. For one, I don't hate women no matter how much pain they have inflicted upon us, I pity them. Hating them would be too easy to do and it would only destroy me and not them. Two, I have been married to my wife of thirty-two years at the printing of this book. She has put me through a lot of the shit I will warn you away from in this book. She has also drastically changed her life not to follow this hateful path of hurting men because she was simply raised that way. So if you are MGTOW with a woman who wants to change I can understand you not running headlong for the door. But even if my wife was not going to stop treating me like some sort of door-mat for crappy shoes then I would have packed my damn bags and got out of there.

Don't fool yourself for one second, if I had to go one more day with my wife treating me the way your woman might be treating you now, she would find herself alone. Three, I have counseled single, and married couples since 1999 and have written several books on the subject of human psychology as it relates to forgiveness and both genders respecting one another. But in one day and one hour, I gave it all up. I gave up my radio career, my TV appearances when I could no longer put a bandage on the hurt and devastation that the Women's Liberation Movement was causing all innocent men.

I didn't immediately become an MGTOW back then, mainly because I didn't even know it existed. I got to admit it is an excellent idea whose time had long been overdue. If the guys who invented the movement had not then I believe I would have. I additionally was given the maximum amount of support by the same woman who caused me so many damn problems in the first place. I guess after she had taken her version of the red pill she awoke too and was feeling remorseful for the hurt she had caused. Today I take on that mantle with every beat of my heart and there is no turning back until the government of each country stops this bull-shit of trial by penis in order to favor vagina.

So, let us get to work, and together we can bring this mess to a grinding halt in less than a year if we get this book around to enough men globally. If we are to make a difference that manifestation must show through us publically and not just rest within our comments in cyber-space. A movement like this, although great at its inception will wither on the vine of great intentions if you don't make it a physical movement. In part of it being a physical movement will require your physical presence and letter-writing campaigns when I ask for it on a moment's notice. That is why I will teach you as we train soldiers in the military how to become one cohesive force for change.

To meld together millions of different men into one cohesive movement takes outstanding attention to detail and an Esprit-de-corps in order to garner political and societal respect.

In whatever country you may find yourself reading this book you have a military force. It is within that force that men have started as many but ended as one. Those men come from all corners of your country by race, creed, and background but they come. Some come to serve a cause larger than themselves as well as some that come to find out what manhood is all about. Now, I don't mean that you have to be a part of any military to be a man because some of our larger heroes have never even worn a uniform.

If I could take you back in time with my military induction; you would have seen the over four-hundred-fifty guys that joined my basic training unit in 1984. We were told by the main Drill-Sergeant in charge that the Army only needed about one-hundred-eighty-five of us and no more. He said it was his job to cut the numbers in front of him virtually in half. I must tell you that by the end of that training he did just that. What had come to basic training on Fort Knox Kentucky was not the same type of person who graduated.

Those guys initially had nothing in the world to connect them as a brotherhood beyond their enlistment in the service of their country. But the Army of the United States has a unique thing they do by taking males from all fifty states and every background in order to make them one cohesive fighting force. They have a motto that goes, "If you sweat together you will stick together." We grew from a loose-knit, rag-tagged bunch of separatist boys that were more for ourselves and our neighborhoods than we ever were for our country of birth.

I believe that this is the same teamwork that has to take place within the MGTOW International community to effect political and social change. We must be one cohesive organization in order to demand any change we wish to see. The "National Organization for Women" did not start as the firebrand institution it is today. Back then they were a very loose-knit group of women without organization and able to affect no change. But just as with soldiers all they needed was a little teamwork and sticktuidness.

After three months of basic training and three months of training on becoming a Cavalry Scout, we too were one cohesive fighting spirit. You couldn't have separated our love for one another in peacetime any more than you would have on the battlefield. So, believe me when I tell you that we have to get our shit in order and start caring about something broader than our individual communities. If not, we are condemning the up and coming little boys to a fate worse than death itself. I can see a time coming without change that every broad sweeping law created is just to curtail our already fleeting freedoms.

If it were not bad enough that they have to legislate our slavery to the female gender as much as we are groomed in our birth homes to serve. The modern female victim song believes that they are the only ones to service husbands and children. But I am telling you long before you could tie your own shoes you were being prepared to be a slave to your wife or girlfriend. As boys, we are raised to grow up and care for a woman as a wife, mother, and sister, whatever. But the one thing a feminine society will never raise a boy to do is to respect his father, himself or his fellow brother. This type of homegrown hatred is the hallmark of the blue pill thinking. In a servitude environment, you seek the respect of the captor in charge of the matrix more than the captive brother.

The way men have sold themselves out over the last generation and submitted themselves to the feminist ideology is equivalent to treason. I am reminded of the British Colonel in the movie, "Bridge on the River Kwai." If you haven't seen the movie yet I highly recommend you do. Anyways, the movie focuses on the officer in charge of losing his mind in a futile attempt to help his Japanese captors dominate his own men. The Colonel only regained his composure and mental faculties once he saw another prisoner of war getting shot before him. It was at that moment that he decided he would blow up the bridge that he had for so long built for his enemy with his soldier's blood sweat and tears.

If you are a man who is new to the MGTOW Movement then I can see why you think this organization is hateful towards women. But this is why the analogy between the blue and red pill is being made. Awakening from a resting state that has been a part of your psyche since your birth is a hard thing to do; in that, you are only challenging your assumptions and beliefs. There is no problem in feeling empathy for women in the world today; the larger problem is when you feel only animosity and separation from your own gender.

As men, most of us wake up without the aid of the red pill after the wedding day has passed or we allow a woman to move into our homes. We wake up to wives arguing incessantly with us or running away from us back to their parents without cause. We snap back to reality after she has either wiped our bank-accounts clean or cut up all of our clothing; we wake up. But if this was our awakening moment then what was the unconscious moment that made you enter this relationship? You broke covenant with reality once you locked eyes with her rear-end and decided you were in love with her ass and not your future. You surrendered to a reality of pain over pleasure when you fell for her breast long before you even looked at her face.

Why do we do this as guys, you might ask? We do this because our masculine brain releases a large amount of dopamine, the pleasure-chemical along with norepinephrine into our circulatory system at lightning speeds. These functions virtually take place without our prodding once we are attracted to someone physically or sexually. The second thing your masculine brain does is shut off what I refer to as the bullshit-guard. The bullshit-guard or the amygdala portion of the brain which is designed to warn us of impending danger or future calamity. The amygdala which is present in both hemispheres of the brain is the body's chief cautionary system since you were a born. It has recorded every foolish attempt at self-sabotage and near-death catastrophes you have performed since you placed your mother's fork in that wall socket. Since you rode your bike with no hands and missed that rock I the street ended up with your arm in a cast.

Another portion of the brain that got disabled once you viewed that girl in lust was your reasoning hemisphere or the frontal lobe. The frontal lobe is the rational center of the brain and it would have told you to stop and check this girl out first. This same frontal lobe that missed her lies this time will return to warn you a couple of years down the same road. If any girl meeting this same girl's criteria image of pain tries to smooth talk you alarm bells will go off. But what do we do, when those alarm bells go off?

We proceed to hit the key-fob quickly enough to dampen the sound so we can get our dicks wet and our lives wrecked in the after crash. You do these enough times and you have essentially taken yourself off of the available market for women. Why? By then you will be as financially broke and broken as a man that no woman would be willing to talk to you anyways. This girl who now causes your mind to sleep but your libido to be aroused would have purchased a lifetime of clothing on your time while you have nothing but high-waters in your wardrobe. You would have exchanged a very short time of pleasure for a long time of suffering.

You will leave that relationship through a divorce with nothing left that you spent years achieving. On the other hand, she will own a world of possessions that she would not have without your hard work and perseverance. This woman that used to live in her mother's basement will have in her possession, your house, your children and your brand-new car in your brand-new finished driveway. The only thing you will have is either a park bench or a homeless community shelter after the local police evict you from that once bachelor-pad. To add insult to injury the court system will mandate that you support her lifestyle in a house you can no longer visit, stay in, or share with your child. A child I might say that she turns against you on a daily basis.

So, starting today you are going to have to know how to go into a room with your mind thinking and not your dick. For it is our dick that talks us into all of these no-good relationships. And it is our dicks that walk away with us as the only property we have from a life of former personal satisfaction. You see when you lose to a woman your property you also lose your self-esteem. You believe yourself to be stupid for allowing the same thing to happen to you that happened to someone in your family past.

From this day forward as long as you are in the presence of sexy women know that you will be out of the presence of mind. You will not be in touch with your capacity to reason as long as you are physically or sexually attracted to a woman in what I refer to as your "weakness-sphere."

The weakness-sphere only triggers with your perception of youth and vigor in the opposite gender. If a woman before you were a ninety-five-year-old you would not have this problem. No, for the ninety-five-year-old woman you would only feel compassion for her age and experience. As men, we are vulnerable in this way because the female gender is our natural sexual partners and not our natural enemies. This gender has only recently over the last fifty-years made itself our foe. The only problem with this thinking is that our dicks never got the enemy mobilization memo.

In the entirety of animal species all males pursue their female equivalent because they are sexually attracted to her and you, my friend is no different. In the entirety of the animal species, the logical mind of each male creature gets turned off, and sometimes to their detriment. They just as you can lose their lives and territories in the pursuit of copulation. Dogs die crossing streets in an attempt to follow the pheromones of a bitch in heat. Birds get so tunnel focused that they can be either eaten by predators or ran over by cars. The praying-mantis gets his head literally eaten off by his mate and I don't have to tell you where the black-widow spider got her name from. And if you remember, you got your ass handed to you messing with too many women because of your dick.

In the complete animal species of female to include humans, they are mainly selfish. Female animals are selfish in that they take care of their birthed progeny more than the male to which that progeny came from. So, for a human woman to love you, she will have to basically rise above herself in order to give you the respect she so richly adores from you. In the entirety of the species female, they always group for protection and friendship. These behaviors are opposite for all human/animal males who typically act as loners in search of female's in a competition for sex and partnership. Unfortunately, the trick that bonds male to female is what he will not get in a relationship with her. Once the romance period has passed, he can say goodbye to his precious sex and close partnership.

Sure, men in their youth like all animals will find a running male partner but they are soon separated once one of those males chooses a mate. You might notice that if you have a friend as an adult male you lose him shortly after you find a mate. Men typically don't want to stand in the way of their buddies starting a brand-new life. And if he didn't walk away happily, your new bride would develop over one-million reasons why you shouldn't hang with him.

This divide-and-conquer attitude of our human female mate is why we have been scattered-brained for over the last forty-five plus years. The worst thing is not that we let it happen; the worst thing is that we are allowing it to happen to every new generation of a little innocent boy. It may be too late for you if you are a grown man. But what of the baby boys? If you fail to act now, he will be groomed to be a statistical failure. From his mother to his teacher and every female in between will be grooming him to be a human ATM machine by the time he arrives at adulthood.

So, I want you to change the way you approach sexuality and attractiveness if you are to become something other than a spineless male for women to abuse. Tomorrow I want you to place yourself around the most attractive woman that you see as your type. I want you to experience what your body is putting you through. I want you to understand that your penis which has no brain is asking you to be poor and broken down the road. Don't worry about what the woman in your presence is doing to turn you on. Sure, she is going to play a sexually attractive game with you even if she doesn't like you because she feels that men are just weak putty in the hands of women.

> *"What you can walk away from you have mastered; what you cannot walk away from has mastered you."*
> Mike Murdock

I don't want you to play with her fire, as your dumb ass has done in the past.

This time I want you to simply walk away. Every occasion you find yourself in the presence of the opposite gender is not a chance to play hide-the-nightstick. When you walk away you choose life over death, wealth over poverty and freedom over bondage. Trust me, I walked away from plenty of women prior to being married to my current wife but even that doesn't guarantee a successful outcome. What it guarantees you is a successful outcome of being in charge of what I refer to as the "Delayed Reflective Mind." The delayed reflective mind exists in all of our psyches and doesn't need you to be sexually aroused to rip you off.

The delayed reflective mind is out for itself and your future be-damned. It is in it for the reward, in ignorance of the punishment. Let me explain to you how it works in order that you can take it under control before it does the same to you that it did to your father. The delayed reflective mind is your consciousness out of whack for just enough time that it takes to get you into a shit-load trouble down the road.

The delayed reflective mind has been with you since the day it encouraged you to lie to your mother in order to get what you wanted or perceived you needed and couldn't. Say as a child, you wanted some monies to buy some junk food for school the next day and your mother said, no. The delayed reflective mind would then encourage you to steal these monies at night; form her purse, believing that she would never miss it.

The next morning, with the booty of change, you nabbed from her purse, you proceed to the store and buy your tasty treats. That afternoon your mother confronts you and tells you that she desperately needed the money you stole. For your misdeeds, she punishes you to your room with no dinner as she says you have eaten already your reward. While in that room, with enough time to look back and reflect on what happened; the delayed reflective mind comes to visit you. Your mind says, "why did you do that to your mother, she is doing all she can to take care of you. See, this is another example of why you are a bad child."

How funny it is when the delayed reflective mind criticizes you for the trouble it prompted you to do in the first place. Similarly, when we are in the range of romantic confrontations with women; it is the delayed reflective mind encouraging us for what it will correct us for later, as we sit in divorce court. You never want to submit your power to any woman. As a man, you would never submit your control to another man. No, in the presence of another man we would either say or think, "You are not going to control me."

So why is it that you would yield your intelligence to a woman that you wouldn't either talk to or give a second glance if it were a male? Are you sure the women you had to rob your life were as crazy as you thought they were or did you suffer from a momentary bout of insanity in their presence? Work on this first lesson for a couple of weeks and you will change your entire life. When you are next in the company of a woman who wants to entice you sexually as a game use this technique.

I want you to see her as what used to be referred to as a "mix-tape salesman." The mix-tape salesman was just a guy in the neighborhood who boot-legged so many songs off the radio or recorded music to resell them as profit. Now sure this was illegal as hell but it didn't stop him from going around bugging people with the tag line, "hey man, I got them mixed tapes."

Most people just turned him down as a nuisance knowing that he would approach them on the next day. See her as the mix-tape salesman, only she has as sex in the place of the tapes. She sees each man as a joke to play a game she does not intend to carry out just for fun. As you see this woman coming from a block away keep in your head, No! I don't want any mixed tapes, leave me alone. For sure she will show offense on her face as she passes you because you neither look at, smile at nor play her game of enticement. She may call you or think of you as gay, but you rather be thought of as gay instead of being broken, busted and grim on the other side of her manipulating game.

What if I am seeking a Beaver or Already Married to a One?

"In order to catch the life saboteur beaver ones mind must first become as sharp as a steel trap."

Charles Rivers

There is certain math about you that has attracted every woman you ever known to your presence or caused her to run for the exit. In order to escape a repetitious matrix of relationship hell, you must first know what attracts these beavers to your inner consciousness.

Without this precious knowledge, men are left to ponder, what in the hell, is wrong, with me? We are left to wonder, why I continue to elicit the same, "love-challenged-beavers" into my life; while effortlessly pushing away the exciting women I desire most. If you are tired of getting the same no-growth, money-draining beaver chicks that just need your couch to crash, simply means that you are sending out erroneous vibes. You are going to have to make a dramatic change in your life signal.

"If you cannot be true to yourself, what challenge does someone in your presence have to be true to you?"

Charles Rivers

As we grow into being adult, working-class persons we take on a persona that is not genuine to our conscious or unconscious psyche. Most males are so far removed from being their best-selves since childhood that even family and loved ones struggle to understand who the hell is this person?

Becoming the Most Original You

All of us live, a real, but different life behind closed doors at home; but this does not have to be. In order for you to enjoy the abundance that life has to offer you, you will have to return to the original you.

If you do not change yourself first, you will continually attract that which you have been trying to avoid. I don't believe in calling people losers, but I do believe that all of us have a spirit that attracts a certain style of woman and continual negative events into our life. After constantly getting this same dry feedback loop day-by-day, we actually believe ourselves to be the people and circumstances that gravitate towards us. But I'm sure that within your life you have seen a hero or romantic movie.

In these movies, the lead character always gets the beautiful knowledgeable and supportive woman of his dreams. Why is that? In each one of those books and movies, I guarantee that you have never seen an opening line that went: *"The Hero is an Outstanding Follower of other Peoples Goals for Himself."* Nope, what you read or seen was that the desired person was an individual with a passion for life, love, and risk-taking. This fantasy is precisely what most men I have met are looking for in other people but simultaneously deny for themselves. All human being is born with a passion for these character traits, but we trade this spirit in for a passion for retirement.

What Kind of Beaver Trap Signals am I Subconsciously Sending Out?

In this exercise in order to consciously attract true love over beaver love, you must be comfortable yourself. In order to be, one, you must first find out, "who am I?" You are more than simply your surface appearance of well-manicured looks, deodorants and smart clothing. What we see in the mirror every morning is definitely not what beavers see in us. These superficial markers that we believe make us appear as the hero escape the notice of those who are attracted to us physically, mentally and emotionally.

An adult males body chemistry may be sending out one three-dimensional image he is trying to project, but his subconscious is making an up or down vote for his relationships at the same time. The subconscious mind is unlike the body and will, block affairs of the heart that conflict with your true aura. People that are interested in us see our unconscious projection of our inner selves long before they see our sexual looks. The beaver in the wild is known as crafty, intelligent, and industrious animal is best known for ingeniously altering its environment. In this case, if you are not powerfully careful your world will be that altered environment.

If you want to know what the Beaver you are trying to attract sees as opposed to what you see in the mirror, stop listening to what your male friends who are poor trappers are telling you.

There is a big difference between what a good friend sees, and what a potential night long, or lifelong Beaver sees. With buddy friendship; like attracts. Like meaning that your buddy is with you because you are quite similar to him in every way. But in love, likeness repels but draws opposite consciousness. Why is this you might ask? This is because the Beavers that are attracted to you see something in your consciousness that is missing within their consciousness. You are similarly attracted to them because they have a strength that is your chief weakness. For example, if you are a closed communicator, you will be attracted to an open intellectual Beaver that may be mouthy.

You are attracted to that Beaver because they have the unashamed spirit to speak their mind, no matter who is listening. They are attracted to you because although you appear strong, you are more subdued and patient in spirit; which is what they wish they truly were. Now both of you may have friends outside of the home that reflects your consciousness and spirit, but this will never complete you as a person. Chief in the spirit of all male maturation is in surviving and thriving through negative people and events that most challenge him. Hence the basic training scenario. For it is where the typical male is blindsided that he lacks all knowledge. A friend can only sharpen the same knowledge, but the opposite gender or untested event can sharpen where you are deficient.

Completion of any spirit, headed towards clarity involves both sides of the brain; and not just the same side you share with your buddy. Sure, opposite sides of the subconscious attract in love; which is why opposites attract but growth occurs when you try to challenge those opposite attractions. Remember, you will attract only what you are missing within yourself, not what you have. So, if you don't want to attract a Beaver who is dead-set on fixing you then, repair yourself first. The second thing that guys ask me is why then do most guys marry women who don't meet a superficial model's appearance?

This is true, typically in a relationship, you will mainly see Beavers getting married that does not meet the made-up standard of beauty. Most of these women will be less than six foot as opposed to the models in the magazine ads and many that look nothing like the airbrushed fashionistas that grace the pages at the checkout counter.

Why is that? Well just like those movies and books I spoke about a minute ago, typically men are attracted to women who need rescuing. Similarly, although women are very capable of taking care of themselves are attracted to tall men who want to look out for their well-being. Women just have a fault in that they try to slay their rescuer so they can be free to be rescued again. The average woman believes as men in the chase and not the capture. So, if you are broken within your spirit, you will attract a suitor, who not only has what you are lacking but sets out to fix that deficiency of brokenness.

So how do we get more of what we want and less of what we don't from Beavers? First, you have to evaluate what repeat signal you are sending out. A minute ago, I told you that most people are not the person they were born to be. Therefore, you are sending out an inauthentic signal and ending up with an inauthentic matching woman. So, get out, and work on yourself and your shortcomings long before you invite someone into your life, or she will show up as a repair-woman with the wrong tools to fix you. If you are searching for an open Beaver, with her own income and the life you desire for yourself then become this type of person.

To Catch a Beaver

In order to catch your particular Beaver, you must think like a Beaver. Beaver traps and bicycles are made out of similar metals. Tomorrow, go to your local bike shop and purchase a brand-new bike for riding and having fun. Find the well-traveled bike trails in your town where the Beavers that you want a real relationship to grow with are hanging out. Start riding your bike there for at least twelve days, without expecting anything; your subconscious mind will do the rest. Sooner or later you will develop a whole new additional set of friends to compliment your current buds. Your new set of friends will yield for you without planning or manipulation a whole new bevy of well-complimented Beavers that meet your desires for love. Why did this happen for you now, instead of in the past?

In the past, you were comfortable in finding a Beaver, at the job, in your community or a place that was typical for you. But if you want to find someone who is not typical in the first place, you will have to go to unusual places. Secondly, you became what you were when you were a little boy again, free! Most compatible gender relationships are attracted to the freeing spirit of each other more than looks or income.

When the Beaver of your dreams saw you doing something that she thought was out of the ordinary for you, she became drawn to you immediately. The new problem you will develop is how to turn away so many new potential suitors. The second thing you will notice is that these new suitors are a cut above the women that used to destroy your life were.

Remember, the suitors did not change, you did. Before, you were a boring person, who was not connecting to the free spirit of the child within you. You were a person who subconsciously was drawn to the domineering ball-crushing spirit that your mother placed over your father. But that was their life and not yours. Remember, I told you at the beginning of this book I feel it my job to either help you get a better relationship. Improve the one you are in or hit the bricks to a better life.

How Do I know if this Beaver is Right for Me?

You will know, almost immediately if she is the right fit for your growth and development based upon your amygdala. If you remember I told you earlier, that the amygdala portion of your brain warns you of impending danger, or situations it deems bad for you. In this case, you can count on if you are attracted to the person; the amygdala will also go off like a sixth sense. In this case, I don't want you to fear, but to drive forward and make a connection in the relationship. You will always have the amygdala going off, not simply for enemies, but also for progress. You see when you want to buy a new car, the amygdala goes off. When you want to buy a new home, start a business or talk to the person of your dreams the amygdala will sound the alarm.

Why does the amygdala do this to us? The amygdala is our warning system not only for failure but success. Your amygdala is saying, your father never achieved these dreams, so you should learn to live down in order to be satisfied. The amygdala warns, your father never did have the model wife in your mom who would support him so you should settle for an average woman to dominate your freedom. Its reasons that you should find a woman who knows what is best for you.

This is precisely the reverse Beaver trap that your father fell into in your mom. How can a woman know what is best for you as a man if she has never spent one day of her life as a male? The call for a wife or a girlfriend or a piece-of-ass as life-guide is nothing more than the call of your mother's voice. The amygdala is only sounding off this alarm because you either do not know this Beaver as yet or you have no experience with climbing higher. Many people in life usually turn back, when they get what is called, a gut-feeling but it is the amygdala that is sending you that feeling. The amygdala starts in the head, long before it shows up as a burning twinge in your gut.

So, if your alarm bells are going off and this Beaver does not pose a clear and present danger to you, then introduce yourself. Most men are afraid to approach the prettiest woman of their dreams on the streets where they find them. But the subconscious has no fear of anything of the conscious mind and it rests within your same wakened body. You have met, kissed and had sex with more beautiful women in your dreams at night than you ever attempted to say hello to in your awakened state. You remember in your dreams you would do this naturally. You would do this without thinking about it in your unconscious state because most inhibitions lie mostly in your conscious state.

Societal inhibitions don't have the authority to penetrate and ruin dreams in the unconscious lucid thinking MGTOW mind that is why you have sex with total strangers in your dreams. That is why you argue with someone or defend yourself heroically in your unconscious state, wherein society you would never do such things. So, the next time you are out Beaver hunting, I want you to do are to have the highest expectations for a new relationship. Like one guy told me once, "MGTOW doesn't mean celibacy for everyone."

Some of the largest relationship killers and arguments come out of low guessed pre-living arrangement expectations. This time, don't let yourself, fall into the trap of not saying what you would desire up front, only to regret it ten years down a broken relationship road with child-support for a platoon-sized group of children. The next time you are out Beaver hunting know that they vary in almost every region you find them; so, fear be-damned. In this case, fear means, that you are on the right track for growth. Comfort means you have peaked that growth.

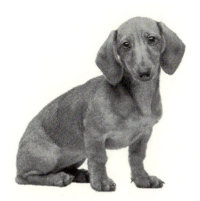

Dachshund Feminist
(The *Victim*)

"The initially cute and lovable Dachshund Feminist has occupied and frustrated more homes and marriages than the angered Radical Feminist will ever be privileged to."

Charles Rivers

The hardest weakness for most men to overcome is that of volunteering to rescue a victim. Whether it is a kid trapped in a running stream, a Dachshund lost from home or a woman who looks to naive to deal with the real world. The only difference between the three categories I just name you is that the woman is purposely acting like a victim in order to have power over her rescuer. For she knows far better than he that only men respond to the false nature of a woman. She could never try and use her feminine-wiles or weaknesses on another woman for her sister would not only know that she is a bull-shitter, but she would call her out for being one.

Honestly, my largest hurdle when introducing men to their

consciousness to be whole men is what they don't know about women.

It took me many years and two decades of counseling to be able to assist guys through the games that women were playing. In this chapter, I am going to try and impart you with as much information on the tricks of the Dachshund Feminist. Before I knew how to disarm the women who brought their unsuspecting husbands into counseling I too was being blind-sided. What you must learn first is that the average female who is trying to pull the wool over your eyes is already guessing twenty steps ahead of you.

That's right, twenty steps. This is why if you get into an argument with a woman you end up losing. She has thought through the argument within the moment and every answer you are going to give back in defense of your actions. In my experience, I can honestly say that women are not any smarter than men when it comes to arguing but how stealthily they approach the discourse. Let me give you an example so you can best resolve any future negative interactions with the women in your manosphere.

One afternoon at my counseling headquarters I was called by a man who had heard my radio show. He wanted to come in and bring his wife for me to mend the brokenness within his home. Upon meeting him that afternoon alone I asked where was his wife. He admitted to me that he wanted to try my counseling first before he brought her in alone. He told me that his profession was that of a television minister and that his name should not be used outside of that room or it would damage his career. I agreed although I have never used anyone's name that was held in private counsel.

He said that she had moved out of their shared bedroom down to his daughter's room at the end of the hallway. He said that she was holding some sort of grudge against him but he didn't know what it was. He informed me that she would not enjoy my company any more than she relished his on meeting me. I asked was it that she disliked males, or what. He said, no, I don't think that is the reason. He said, you are just going to have to ask her yourself.
After lengthy one-sided counseling that afternoon I departed him

with a game-plan on how was I going to approach this wife of a church pastor.

True-to-form once she arrived the next day she looked as if she had no love for me. She shook my hand with the cold fish handshake and took a seat. Along with my stenographer, I offered her refreshments along with a catered meal. She refused both and said she just wanted to get this over. She said she was here merely because her husband wanted her to be here. At that moment I told her that I didn't want her in my office for that reason and that she could leave anytime she was ready, with her husband's money for this session.

She said, no, I'll stay. She said that she was intrigued to meet whomever her husband was raving about fixing his outlook on life in one afternoon. She said I have never seen anyone change his responses to life. I told her that I was hoping to do the same for her. The reason I left counseling many years later because I was not in it for the money but for the change and mending of lives. I asked her, what made her move out of her shared bedroom with her husband? Was it that she believed he had been unfaithful? She said, no, he knows what he did. You see fella's; here is the point in which the counseled person is beginning to try to lead the counselor.

Here is the point in which the woman in your life is trying to rout you through a maze of twenty-questions. Don't take the bait any more than I would have. I asked the preachers wife, is there anything I can do to help you mend this relationship? She said, not really, I would be glad just to live down the hall in my daughter's room. You see it was at this point that she was beginning to lead me into asking her about her daughter but again, I didn't take the bait. So, I changed the subject and began to set up my own trap for the Dachshund Feminist. I asked her, so mam, what do you like doing in the church?

She said I like helping the couples at our church and I enjoy baking cookies for them. Ironic isn't it that people are usually very successful at the things they fail very miserably at home. This for me gave a change direction two as I knew continuing down any one particular path would have us there for days of misdirection. I said so you being the wife of a Christian Pastor you are pretty familiar with the four Greek Biblical Loves. For those of you who are also unfamiliar with the original definitions of love where I give you the names here.

You have Eros Love, Philia Love, Storge Love, and Agape love; with Agape being highest. I will explain each after I complete the story for you. But I will preface it by saying that all four loves were replaced in today's dictionary with simply the word, "love." But love does not go far enough to describe all of these varied truths of love.

The preacher's wife revealed to me honestly that she only had a vague understanding of two of the definitions but she knew what Agape Love was. So, I took my time to set up the moment that I was going to shut-down her charade show at hurting her husband while baking cookies for strangers. If you the reader can grasp these love levels you will also know why you may have never truly experienced real love over false love or just sex. Many men raised by an unloving mother have no clue how love should act or feel. And if you are looking to get into a relationship with a woman without the knowledge of these four you are really setting yourself up for a good old-fashioned ass-whooping.

Back then I used to begin all of my seminars with this quote of mine below. If you are married or unmarried you may still question yourself for the answer as we work our way to understanding the Dachshund Feminist. I asked the preacher's wife this same question at this point.

"Why is it that a typical friendship is capable of lasting twenty years or more while a marriage is hard-pressed to last barely two years?"
Charles Rivers

So, let's take it from the top. The basic, bottom love level is **Eros Love** or what you refer to as erotic love. Eros love covers everything sexual or romantic. If you watch xxx porn movies then these are known as erotic movies. If you know of a woman who is heavily into fantasy novels and films then this too is Eros love. To be sure Eros Love covers every relationship to where you chose the physical beauty and the body over substance in a relationship. Most people, worldwide are let the fuck down when they awake the next morning after screwing someone for an erotic fulfillment only. This is why you ask a woman to leave your house and never call you again.

Worse still is most men tried to form a relationship over a lifetime based upon the initial sexual or physical attraction. These relationships suffer the most and gain no traction for both of the participants. Why, because Eros Love is no more than a bodily function like wasting in the toilet. I bet you didn't see that coming. Yes, it is a function or an urge that has really nothing to do with love. Let us go sideways for a moment and talk about urges so you won't fall for another hollow relationship again in your MGTOW life.

You see without true love from a woman to a man the relationship is little more than a bodily function. As in food is desire to eat, your bladder full is a desire to pee, and your bowels remind you of the need to pass excrement. You may also answer the call of horniness by manipulating yourself to orgasm by masturbation, internet porn or by abstaining.

But you could never abstain from food, water, urination or wasting without dying. So, although we think that we would die without sex we are actually fooling ourselves because this is a hollow desire with no consequences, not even blue-balls to which we will talk about later in the book. I made sure the preacher's wife understood this loving level before moving on. I also explained to her how she was failing at it by being at the end of the hall from her husband and not in her bed where she promised him on the alter, she would be. I feel if you hold back something as small as sex how will you deal with something as large as cancer?

The next love level from the bottom was, **Philia Love**. Philia Love is what is known as friendship love. It is a love you can experience with your best friend or your mate. I find that teaching on this subject for over two-decades that no couple makes it long term without Philia Love. The name is so powerful that it is part of the city name Philadelphia or, "The City of Brotherly Love." Under Philia Love you have done some of the most enjoyable to heinous acts with your best buds and women have done the same with their girlfriends. The only problem is that both genders have not accorded the same pleasures they extend to their same-sexed friends to each other.

Philia Love requires no sex or romance but all communication. Philia Love is the only love that is optimal for a lifetime relationship to last. If you look back at all of your lasting or memorable relationships in life, they all existed above the belt and not below it. Sex in and of itself does not endear a person to you for any length of time. If I ask you to think of your childhood friend and something stupid you guys did together a smile would come to your face. They could have gotten you in trouble back then and you could very well forgive them as being just young. You could have separated in a negative way but you still have fond memories of your time together.

I explained to her that she was not a friend to her husband by alienating her above the waist love by living down the hall. Once she understood the gravity of Philia Love I asked her to answer this second question for me that I had pioneered for difficult couples.

"If my spouse was my best friend in the world right now, would I be able to get away with treating them the way I do now, or would I have to change?"

Charles Rivers

This brought us to the next level of love or, **Storge Love**. Storge Love is the love that parents have for their children as they try to fold them into the already existent love within the home. Without Storge Love, the child has nothing to base his love when raising their own children. A mother who has an absence of Storge Love prefers to exchange the love of career over the love of a child. In her estimation, everything and everyone in her home must fall a distant second to her personal, professional and selfish pursuits in the world.

This is why feminism itself is one gigantic selfish pursuit for women. Ask yourself, why would a single woman who claims to hate men be marrying one. In fact, why would a single woman who claims to hate men, marry one and have a baby by the same. What about having a baby by the man you hated marrying then hating the baby you created together.

The only thing that is more insane than the previous three is loving the child that came from the man more than the man himself. How do you derive love from hate? At no time should Storge Love take away from the love that both parents have for one another? Remember, Storge Love, folds the child into an already existent love or existent hate. I explained to the Dachshund Feminist, better known as the preacher's wife that she was damaging the Storge Love in the home by bringing her innocent daughter in the middle of the hell she had created between her husband and her.

Now it was time to close and nail this coffin shut on a woman who had come in my office with a grudge against her husband. I had been waiting for this last and top level of love since I started the conversation with her but I had to cover everything from the bottom first. As the reader, I hope you understand up to this point, why the simple modern word love cannot take the place of these different categories of love. By now, you probably understand more why most of the encounters you had with women were not as loving as you thought they might have been.

This brings me to the final level of love or, Agape Love. Agape Love is the highest of human loves and it lends itself to what the Greeks called the love that God for man and that man should extend to his fellow brother. In essence, anyone who calls themselves as loving God, going to a church of any denomination or who has a personal relationship with their creator. You see I went this route with her because she was a preacher's wife. I needed to stray with her away from traditional counseling if I was to beat her at the game of twenty and have her make any sort of change.

I said to her mam; now that you are familiar with all four love levels let me ask you one final question. Do you love God? She said, "oh yes I do, with all of my heart." The bait was out fella's and I had the rabbit in the entrance of the cage. As she sat at the table to which I counseled her nearer to the stenographer I asked her my last query. I got up from that table and went to stand under the beam of a bright light that streamed from the ceiling.

I placed both of my arms ceiling-ward towards the bright light and asked just this. Mam, how can you then hold your loving arms up to God in Agape Love and say I love you Father; turn those same arms towards your husband and say, I have no love left for you.

She immediately got up and ran out of my office. I was left awestruck. Was it something I said? Did I go too far even with a religious woman? I was sure I would hear back from her husband in a couple of days how she had hated my counseling and how I had failed miserably as a counselor to convince her to be better with the guy she swore on an altar to be better with. True to form on the afternoon of the next day her husband showed up to my office with a check for the counseling. He told me we are finished. I said was it something I did that your wife didn't like?

He said, "on the contrary, you did an excellent job." He said, "I don't know what you said to her and I don't have to know." What I do know, is she came to the car crying, sat down and didn't say anything all the way back home. As I sat downstairs of our home, I heard her making clambering sounds upstairs for hours. Thinking she was going to leave me faster after you talked to her, I didn't get involved. When everything finally fell silent, she came down the stairs. She came in front of me and apologized for acting the way she had been acting.

She told me how much she loved me and that she defiantly had not been showing me, love. That entire racket she had been making was her moving her stuff back in our room. If I ever get a couple in my counseling and I can't turn them around as quickly as you turned my wife back into my arms, I'm calling you. After listening to your radio show I knew that if anyone could turn our relationship around or help us to go our separate ways it would be you. So, you see my MGTOW brothers if you have not been receiving but sex from the women you have known over a lifetime then you have never really been in love. Worse than that you have been having sex with women that hated you which is equivalent to paying for sex from a prostitute.

As men, we have a most pitiful tendency to fall hard in love with the feminine weakness of the Dachshund Feminist.

What this usually gets us is a rabid pooch with sharpened claws waiting to strike at our exposed groin. Most men are usually shocked, confused and amazed how quickly misses peace-loving soft-spoken victim becomes a bitch out of hell. But this is usually something we bring upon ourselves. Men are simply attracted to being the rescuer of the victim pooch or damsel in distress. We are secondly attracted to what is missing in our own psyche or personality and lastly, we are attracted to our mother's personality super-imposed on our future mate. I will seek to clarify the three by first attacking your need to rescue a woman who doesn't appreciate your help.

In my classes, I used to explain this concept to the women who attended more than the husbands but today I extend this same advice to you. This "Rescue the Damsel" in a relationship; although cute in the beginning grow old for the woman who doesn't feel like she needs fixing. Additionally, it wears thin on the man who feels like he has already rescued his lady by wedding her out of the evil clutches of her witch-mother in the castle.

What goes over most males' heads once they fall too hard in love with a woman, they believe to be a victim is her experience. I don't mean simply her mental acuity but the fact that she was already an adult when you met her. When you met her not only was she not a waif or a child but she was fully mature. By your introduction she had with her mother's training learned how to use the bathroom on her own. She had learned how to open and close doors for herself and she was pretty good at cooking meals for herself and her house guest. She could drive a car on her own and make a living out of her own education. Then why was it that she decided to be an infant once you took her into your home. From that day until your life fell apart you were being played.

Women are keen at choosing you, long before you believe you have eyed them. After that, it is they who will act accordingly to pull out the nurturer in your spirit in order for you to drop your guard and submit to their will.

If a woman is to use a man, he must act in the role of father to daughter rather than a husband to wife. Playing this game for both is what leads to a woman cheating around on her man. Once a woman places a man in the all-protective fatherly role, she sees him as someone not to have sex with. Although women are just as nasty mentally as men, they do not have father fetishes in a live-in situation.

Not only will you slowly trend to a sexless coupling but you are being trained to be tortured. Once she has you as father/protector you couldn't possibly argue back at her without her crying like your daughter. The money you have to spend on this type of woman is equivalent to a dowry a father owes just to thank you for marrying his daughter.

If you don't give her the monies, she pleads for in a childlike victim voice she will also withhold natural affection from you just as she would a father. So, if you insist on going into a relationship with any woman and you want to be sure not to lose your financial or mental shirt then do this one thing. Allow her to remain an adult and allow her to pay the bill s whenever possible. Yes, even in a live-in situation.

You will need this if you are either put out of the apartment you are renting or removed from your home by the police. As a modern-day man you must do just as women by documenting what she pays versus what you pay. There is not a court in the land that would agree to strong alimony of you paying everything if you only paid part of everything.

They must know that she not only had a history of co-paying the bills but she had the ability to take care of herself before you met and after. Typically, what men do is take over all of the bills and utilities. Once you do this the average woman will retire to that couch and not show her head until you get a divorce. She would have chosen the legal time and date with ample receipts from your knight-in-shining-armor activities in order to fleece your future earnings.

But what if you had let her remain an adult? Even if she burnt her copies of the checks along with her credit card statements this stuff is permanently in these companies' databases. You could easily have your divorce attorney subpoena these documents to support your case. The same should go especially in the case of your children being a babysitter.

In no instance should you pay the entire bill with your bank account? If your wife or girlfriend believes you should then you have a liberated captive woman. In this last instance be very cautious. If you don't learn anything ensure that she pay her own way when it comes to her child. If she had a child by another man before she met you then you don't want the court to believe that you have assumed all of the duties of the absent father and the absence of the mother bills.

If you mistakenly do this when you guys are lovey-dovey with each other and you separate then this child will be your financial responsibility for the foreseeable future. I say child but today there may be many children along with the one you had with her. Feeling sorry for her situation won't feel as empathetic when you receive a garnishment of all of your paychecks until they grow up. Any woman in my book that is willing to let the last guy go and milk a new guy just because he is decent has my vote.

…Moving right along. Let's talk now a bit on the second reason why we rescue absolute total strangers just because they are female.

Most Men Have Unfinished Business with Their Mother's

Most of us leave our mothers about the age of eighteen-years with a bit of remorse and pity for our behaviors under her care. The only time there is an exception to this is if she did not do right by us or she treated our fathers too harshly. This feeling of guilt is the largest feather in the cap of any woman liberated or otherwise. Woman has the tendency to exploit our guilt for our moms and we allow it without knowing. If you lived in a home where your father abused or argued with your mother you feel it is your solemn duty never to argue with or touch a woman. The woman in the relationship has no promise to make about not hurting you while blaming it on her emotions.

If your mother raised you while struggling financially the entire time you feel it is your duty to never let your girl know what poverty feels like. You have assigned yourself as her financial knight-in-shining-armor. She, on the other hand, has no reservation on how your finances turn out. She understands your history, and she, will take every advantage of using your finances as a means to enrich her pocket and wardrobe.

Try to remember what I told males and females alike in my classes. "You cannot fix the future with the past. This is why most children grow up under-nurtured in the care of mothers with husbands. It is because mothers feel that the income that is coming in the home belongs to her solely. She will most assuredly quit her job if you apply the means to struggle for two instead of just yourself. While she's at it she will more than likely get pregnant because if you can take care of two, surely you can take care of three?

Take real caution when getting in any of these types of relationships by leaving whatever you did before you left home between you and your mother and not you and your future son's mother. Most boys that grow up liking their mothers can easily extend that love to their wives but most women who loved their dads; just loved their dads only. She will extend you no courtesies that she would have her father unless her mother was either mean or abusive to her father. In some cases, she might be mean and abusive to you in carrying on her home's demonic legacy.

If you believe you failed your mother in some way before you left home then don't make that up to your girl/wife. If you want to make it up to somebody then your mother will do. But any real mother, worth her salt knows that once a child has left a home that they owe her nothing. She understands that her child was born with a free will that once challenged by her authority was bound to be tested.

Most Men are Missing what their Woman Has

I have been counseling couples for well over two decades now, and I can tell you with relative ease that men unknowingly are chasing what they are lacking. This portion of the damsel rescue is the most dangerous for you. I am sure you have heard of the old adage that opposites attract. But have you heard of the other portion of that statement that says and then they divide? Why do opposites attract? Opposites attract because you see something in that person that you do not possess in your person. For example: If you are a stodgy neat freak who has his life in meticulous order than you may be attracted to a woman who is a scatter-brained hoarder.

Initially, you will find it funny or cute that you have to help her order her life, but this will wear thin rather quickly. Up front, you will find it funny that she lines all of the walls of your house with bags from department stores in her zeal to make you pay for anything on their shelves. Funnier still are most of these packages will remain completely unopened as this is what women call retail therapy. You will find out what you let in your home is nothing more than the death of you for the life of a new matrix. It matters not if you had the conversation with her prior to moving in that you want to keep your place clean. Women have been trained to lie to the men they live closest to and for that reason she will make you the promise that she does not intend to keep.

As I said before due to the fact that the new matrix of filth has taken over your home you must die along with your possessions. I can't tell you how many times I have seen a guy's life erased to make way for the foolishness of a woman he has taken in on the spur of the moment for a piece of ass.

I will give you one sad story in which I knew of three military helicopter pilots that shared a home together. This place was bachelor-pad central with all of the accouterments that men enjoy. But as the years went on, they became civilians and moved to separate homes. The lead guy enjoyed a great bachelor pad with one of his other buddies equipped with a bar and pool table in the basement. We knew that when he came home from a hard day's work, he didn't mean to go to bed stressed out. For two years those guys lived and enjoyed splitting the rent in that bachelor pad until one of the guy's girl-friends moved in.

Of course, you know what happened next. Things in the house began to take on a more feminine design. The male matrix of the home began to be adjusted for the new matrix of pretend wife. In his bathroom where only shaving cream normally, laid items were now positioned and began to smell like lavender. His bathroom in a short time had a complete makeover as if someone exploded a pink bomb in it. Less than a year later he married that woman and sent his friend packing to a place of his own. Now the shit began to hit the fan. That new woman of his sold that bar in the basement and listed the pool table for sale in order to make that a family room.

She moved anything male out of the house and bought a bunch of new furniture with his money as if the house was being staged for sale. She placed cookbooks in the kitchen and on the counter in case her girl-friends showed up. Now, she couldn't cook a lick but that wasn't important as looking as if she was making a nest out of what she believed was his rats-nest. Each time I was over that house more of the life was being drained from him. There was hardly a room where some form of crystal bowl or nick-knack was not being staged.

Finally, the last nail was placed in his coffin when she got pregnant in less than a year of living with him. She quit her job and made a home-office in the basement where his pool table used to rest. She took the extra room in which he used to call his home office and made it the baby's room. So, in less than one year that guy's life had been dramatically erased.

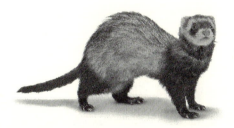

Weasel Feminist
(The *Brainwasher*)

*"The Weasel Feminist is a disease upon innocent relationships.
she wiggles her way into the lives of innocent women
to drive them to hate men just for entertainment."*

Charles Rivers

Most males start out in love completely clueless to what is going to happen even two years down the road in their lives. They dismiss all good advice from other friends and family members about leaving certain categories of no-good women alone. But we do these fruitless things for one of two reasons. The first being that when we choose a woman we are at the height of sexuality in our lives and rebellion. In this mode, correcting a man's decisions on anything is akin as making him stick to that thing.

Do you remember the time in which friends warned you away from getting with the woman that may have ruined your life? Do you remember how they told you that this woman was not right for you and you old them that they were just jealous of your happiness? Do you also remember how you felt once she walked out on you without a moment's notice how ashamed you were?

What of the call you had to make that day to your best buddy in whom you had to swallow a little crow and tell him he was right? What about the other call you made to your parents when you asked them could you move back home because she had just wiped out your bank account? I will go no further, but with these, what if your questions could virtually go all day.

In this chapter, I am going to tell you how to avoid, disarm or take out of commission the Brainwasher Feminist. For she is the most cunning and conniving woman of all. She doesn't approach your home until you date, marry or sleep with another woman. She shows up as liberator to the women in your life with a litany list on why they should hate all things men embodied in you. What she neglects to tell your girl is that she would screw you if her back was turned.

The second reason we choose a woman who is flat-out, no fucking good for us is that we have been trained to love all things feminine and hate all things masculine. Once we are groomed in this mindset, we bring our monies, support, and love home like good little boys. What we get for that in return is disrespect, disdain, and little annoyances. We stick with these relationships the most instead of leaving because our self-esteem is so low that hateful women look like they love to us.

But wait, where did your low self-esteem come from? It came from the women that raised you and was polished to perfection by you. You see the Brainwashing Feminist has been around since you were born. She was the woman who told your mother to watch out because all males are no good. She is the woman who told the girls you dated that you were no good. Finally, she is the one that your girl now calls a friend. Guess what she is saying behind your back. But how do you as a MGTOW be honest with yourself enough to admit that your self-esteem is so low? Because if you can't do this then I can't help you raise it. If you see where you are in life as the be-all and do-all of your existence then you are done. Close the casket, this guy had a good run and his life counted for less than he would have truly known.

In every case where a man has joined the MGTOW Movement, we are dealing with some form of low or lowered self-esteem. Either where a woman took everything that he held as important or she brow-beat him enough to where he is questioning his own masculinity. Well, let me tell you something guys, reduced self-esteem has everything to do with your state of mind if you doubt your masculinity. Hell, even if you are a woman with low self-esteem it is in part because you doubt your ability to be whole as a woman.

Let's have your first self-esteem building class right here and now. I am going to uplift your masculinity about sixty-five percentage points by the time you finish reading these upcoming paragraphs. I use this information to pass onto parents dealing with young boys that have lost their drive to learn based upon the erroneous belief that all boys are stupid and all girls are smart. Again, a belief in the mind of any person usually becomes more real than actual fact. If you were a wee little-boy I could tell you that Santa Claus was going to come down the chimney on Christmas and leave you presents for being good. What I left out was that you lived in a city apartment complex behind a locked door with no chimney.

But what happens after you get old enough to rationalize this is a façade? You grow is what and you proceed to differentiate truth from fiction. As an adult, you get children of your own that you teach this same concept of Santa even though you know it is false. That is why I am telling you now that the people who taught you to place all women on a pedestal and yourself in the basement were wrong. Yes, the same people that taught you innocently about Santa told you to be nice to women. They never told you to which length to take that niceness. They didn't tell you as they informed her to walk out on a man if he wasn't doing the things you wanted him to do or say.

They didn't tell you like they told her to save money for a marriage exit. To keep a bag ready in order to be able to run. Yes, my friend only one gender was listening when they told you, till death do you part and it wasn't women. In knowing this I want to take you back to the little boy you were in order to remove that slave-mentality bullshit from your psyche.

I want you as a MGTOW, to have the ammunition you need for the next time any woman on the street or in your home tells you that all men are stupid. That re-education starts with the road of de-education of Santa Claus beliefs. Additionally, I want you to understand that as an adult male it is our civic-duty to uplift all boys no matter where we find them or the condition, we find them in. The greatest weapon the Feminist Movement introduced was uplifting girls for the future and putting boys down. Over the remaining pages of the chapter, I am going to show you how to educate your male son and yourself from the beginning.

I say to you adamantly that every time you witness a little boy falling short of his dreams and goals; you are viewing his parent's unguarded mindset made flesh upon the world. But don't get it twisted; I am not implying for one moment that his parents purposely wanted him to fail out of life. To the contrary, I am saying that their very direct involvement in the success of his life immensely contributed to which he came to understand. When a parent fashions their life-plan to a boy without his natural abilities secured to those goals you have a recipe for melt-down.

Little boys for the most part up until the age of five years learn primarily from mimicry and through the unconscious actions of their parents and siblings. So, it is expected that when children fail in life it is through the conditionings and lessons learned through those mimicry channels. Most of us want only the best for the children that we enroll in the public-school system for the first time each year but this "best" does not always materialize. Many times, parents are miffed and confused as to why their little boy struggles in school while other children his same age excel.

It pains the average parent to even begin to send that little one off to the world by himself. They fear that maybe they didn't prepare him well enough to compete on his own. But even if that were true, we could only expect him to fail in the same areas the parents struggled in. Why is this you might ask? Because as parent's we teach our boys how to improve at what we failed at as opposed to what they will. We passively taught when we vocalized the words, "I am not good in math, and nor has anyone ever been in our family." So, the first thing we need to do on the road to a healthier and happier school student is clean up and clear out the undermining statements we utter in his presence.

For the very day, he comes to take his teary-eyed seat in the first grade with every bit of separation anxiety the last thing he will need to do is overcome a lack of perceived preparation. Only a few short years of the separation anxiety moment he will be summoned by the teacher to the front of a classroom.

"Go to the chalkboard and write what I tell you down," she says. This beckon forward to the heart of the imperfect boy elicits a wince as the class focuses on his already shivering body and imperfect thought processes. What he will not realize at this moment is that he like so many of the world's greatest inventors was already endowed with greatness before they were fully formed in their mother's womb. Only if he knew that anything he sought to solve, invent, or tackle could be released within the gritty dust of that simple piece of chalk he wields in his hand like an overburdened sword.

What if boys and men like you knew that everything of international significance that was ever invented started in that same wavering mind he possesses. Those same thoughts and inventions were nurtured through this writing instrument. When motivating a little one to what is best within him keep this in mind as you introduce him to learning at home prior to school. A simple piece of chalk in the hands of a wondrously thinking little mind can either be filled with creative inspiration or plain calcium carbonate. As a parent, I must challenge you to go out and purchase a wall-mounted chalkboard with all the accouterments before you get started reading this book.

If your son's school uses a dry erase board this substitute will also work fine. What you would ultimately like to do at this point is to get him acclimated to the same working tools that he would be expected to see in the classroom. If he is already in school these items will just serve as a booster to his support system. Before you begin to use this board with him, first prepare yourself mentally before you prepare his future. You should at no time train him in an angered, frustrated or superior fashion. If you come off in either of these styles of teaching, you will guarantee that he will fail once he comes upon these same items throughout his school tenure.

Ensure that you place that chalk piece you purchased in an ordinary freezer bag so it is visible enough to be displayed on the wall but high enough where he cannot reach it. Allow him and yourself two days before you start this new course. What I want you to do in the mean-time are to learn for yourself and teach him about the magic that is stored-up for the user of this mystical piece of chalk.

He should not casually flaunt the power of the magical chalk piece and its awesome ability to create. If you build up enough anticipative momentum to the power of the chalk within those two days, I guarantee he will show you what magic he sees in its compressed body. You see chalk has been used in countless drafting boards, scientific classes, construction planning and even by such notables as Albert Einstein himself. But you don't have to be an Einstein to produce in three-dimensional space what you write one-dimensionally.

That little dreamer that the school system so casually refers to as a class-clown was born with all of the right ingredients to make his dreams come true. His gifts if truly actualized will benefit humanity far beyond anything you and I can imagine. The problem is that most educators see small boys as something to change rather than someone with a different skill-set than girls. As his parent, you need nothing more for the instruction I teach you here other than what you showed up with. Over the course of coaching couples and individuals in my career, I find the largest hurdle is what you already know.

I tell you the only thing you will have to actively remember is dropping most of what you have learned about teaching and especially concerning boys. As his parent, you are the original programmer to his computer brain and are therefore the only persons who could reprogram that brain by pulling out erroneous or self-damaging input.

Boy's problems and challenges are typically nothing more than mindset changes. In knowing that, you can't change what you can't target and you can't target what you refuse to change. To clear out his negative mindset blockages to superior learning you will have to find out the following things. Whom does he love, whom does he hate? Whom does he respect, whom does he disrespect? What is his fondest dream compared to his worst failing fears? Now let me give you the best example of nature imitating life ever performed in a real-world experiment.

The Flea Experiment

In an experiment, a scientist placed a bunch of fleas in a Mason jar to which the fleas jumped out immediately. The scientist quickly gathered them up and placed the fleas back in the jar, but this time they placed a lid on the jar. The fleas jumped again, but they hit the lid of the jar. After a time to avoid the pain of hitting a closed lid, the fleas began to jump just short of that lid.

The scientist allowed the glass jar to remain undisturbed for one week. After a week had elapsed the scientist opened the lid, and they noticed that the fleas refused to jump beyond where they had been punishingly trained. In fact, they poured the jar of fleas out on the ground and they noticed something totally astonishing. They noticed that these fleas although free never again jumped any higher than the lids distance of that jar from the ground.

In life, if you have gone through a childhood pain or trauma, you may impose your own glass jar ceiling heights onto your child without knowing it. Most of us are simply walking around with imaginative levels of success in which we will not pass in fear of getting hurt. In effect, we are living in a Mason jar of our own making. Unless you learn how to forgive some of your past issues you may be in danger of limiting the Einstein in your imperfect boy. Unforgiven anger is like wearing cement shoes for the most competitive marathon of your life. There is a way to make a difference for wherever there is a problem there is a solution for that problem. In a very recent experiment scientist repeated the flea experiment but this time they did it with a twist that will surely help you and your little boy.

After leaving the fleas in the jar for a week they removed the lid. Sure enough, they noticed the same results of the fleas not jumping beyond the lid. Adjacent to the original flea jar they placed another jar full of fleas in which they mimicked only part of the original experiment. They placed fleas in the jar without placing a lid on the jar. The fleas, of course, jumped out immediately. They recaptured all of the fleas and returned them to a lidded jar. Then they took one flea out of the original short jumping jar and placed it in the new jar with the relatively new fleas. Now here is where science meets life. At once they removed the lid and watched in amazement that when all of the new higher jumping fleas exited the jar, so did the older short jumping flea.

This experiment proves just as with humans if taken out of an old community or Feminist mindset that is limiting to males, you can go and grow higher. Understand that wherever you are in life is wherever you have allowed yourself to imagine. All change occurs from within first and is then manifested on the outside of you. Anything less than that can be faked but not for maximum results. If you want to see a change in his behavior you are going to have to be that change. Grab tightly ahold of his little hand and jump. Jump beyond the limitations of the pains that have restricted your personal, professional and emotional growth. To see results beyond the flea jar of his youthful limitations will only take three days to start.

Re-educating Imperfect fleas: Day 1

There is truly mysticism to the power of a wand of chalk that even a traditional magic wand does not possess. For even a magic wand once waved produces no magic beyond parlor tricks. But it is in the wand of chalk that you can produce anything from the Space Shuttle to colonies on Mars. To wield its gritty power in the hands, of a creative mind can yield you the design for the Empire State Building or the engines for Warp Speed in some far-off distant future.

In this little imperfect boy's hands, you will be shaping a future that you may never be able to witness. We already know that Bill Gates mother never anticipated him making the modern-day programming system, known as Microsoft Windows. So, we can say it was a sure bet that his great, great grandparents never anticipated this force of a boy emanating from their lineage. So, when you teach the former Imperfect boy, I want you to think long term and not just to his adult years.

If in your family history you did not as yet claim a Bill Gates doesn't mean that you will not strike it famous with your son. As a parent or teacher, you have the ability to either reverse a family curse or strengthen it beyond repair. Knowing this, you want to choose the words and actions you use around this new way of teaching wisely. Your actions will either make him live pro or against his own upbringing; prepare him for a mansion or homelessness on a park bench.

After you have permanently placed the chalkboard on the wall and affixed the magical chalk in its rightful place begin to teach. If you teach his mind in a new arena he will never be bored. He won't try to look over your shoulder at the television or outside as a better place to be rather than stuck in your face. You are going to teach on that inspiring chalk piece and the inventors that have gone before him to produce from brain to chalk to board. It is within this golden hour of education that you must sell yourself as a great storyteller. I want you to pull out all of those old hidden inspirational emotions you use to inspire the non-imaginative people of life with.

This you will have to become a success at before he can truly believe in himself or the power of the chalk. As I have said before you have all you need within your person to be successful at training him, because if you didn't have everything you needed then why was he sent to you by the universe? In my many teachings, I have found out that if someone is to fail in life it will only be something that they are already good at. This is true, if you are a motivator at work you will not be at home. The average guy who mows a lawn for a living has the highest grass at the house. So, it is I am sure that in your position within your career you have a knack of motivating people who want to quit sometimes.

To motivate him to inventors within this century and not the last, look up and lean on the talents of those you know will spark his newfound interest to grow. I will give you approximately five names here that tickle the fancy of any little boy. Ensure that your first day's training does not go beyond one hour so you leave his imagination inspired as he goes to play afterward.

Additionally, the human brain of a child makes new connections in its conscious states as well as why he is sleeping. He will dream imaginatively and awake the next day with a new reality beyond his initial limiting beliefs. When he gets up the next morning, he will find that piece of chalk on the wall before you mention it but don't let him use it before the third day.

Famous Inventors of the 20th & 21st Century

1. Robotics — Mr. George Devol
2. Video Game Console — Mr. Gerald A. Lawson
3. Color Television — Mr. Guillermo Camarena
4. The Drone — Mr. Nikola Tesla
5. Dump Trucks — Mr. Robert LeTourneau
6. YouTube — Chad Hurley, Steve Chen, Jawed Karim

Re-educating Imperfect fleas: Day 2

Day two of this new odyssey of learning should take place out of the house. This is the day to take him to the museum so he can see the inventions that came from the same chalk that was once held by little men like him. These inventions that we take for granted today were not always within arm's reach as we have it today. Each one of these guys had a normal father just as you might find yourself today. You do not have to be a rocket scientist mom to inspire your son to be one. It matters if rocket propulsion is your current career, he will simply be inspired because you care for him and the inventions that will wreck your home over the coming years.

The greatest part of this bringing inventions to life day will start right after you leave the driveway. I want to give you all of the power and energy you will need to train your son as opposed to all the bad complaints concerning boys in the 21st century. Boys are not stupid; I say again, boys are not stupid. Far from it, I can remember one conversation with a woman who carried a very terse dislike for her husband and men as a whole. She came into the fancy department store I worked in as a shoe salesman in my youth. She let out insult upon insult about her husband and ending off by looking at me and saying, "but you know how stupid men are?" She did not mind a bit, to include me in on the insult.

I could have chosen to go off on her if I was that type of person. But I didn't, although I wanted to. I stood there for a brief moment thinking about how my wife and children would have to eat mayonnaise sandwiches for dinner if I got fired by responding in kind to her attack. But here is what I said. I said, yes mam, I know exactly what you mean about men being stupid. ***They cut down the forest in this country from coast to coast to build cities by hand. They every road in between and the inventions none of us can do without. Finally, they made this building to include the air conditioner we are enjoying today.*** Yes, mam, I know exactly what you mean about those stupid men. With this she walked away, unharmed but learning that everyone doesn't like sexism, no matter the gender.

I have my entire life been against sexism on both sides of the chromosomes but nothing irks me as hurting males in order to uplift females. You have little girls being raised to think that their male classmates are somehow stupid because they were born with a penis. The largest damage done is one day these young girls will grow up to be the bosses of the men they believe to be stupid. I ask you; how far do you think a female boss would be willing to consider hiring a man that she felt was completely stupid?

Boys today are made to believe that they are stupid because they do not know how many inventions have been made by people who were once their age.

As you ride to the museum, **I want you to ask him to point out something that a boy turned man did not invent.** You can stop at any time within the trip and google that item and the inventor and you will find in short order that everything around you was invented as a solution to a problem; and that it was that little boy who gave his parents an awful time who invented it. Now, this is not sexism, this is fact.

Now I know there will be many people that will be wondering why I chose men to motivate in this book over both genders. My reason for doing so is because if I didn't, I believe I would go to my grave as a failure in this lifetime, despite all I had previously done. Never before in the history of all of mankind, has little boys and men been so vilified, marginalized, maligned, and yet so misunderstood. The average male child beyond the age of infancy is seen as something that is a potential danger to his female counterpart. But in making the human male the national poster-child for re-training we have caused a new problem.

Because of this style of thinking parents have been encouraged to reeducate, medicate or at the very least be careful with young men in public. I don't know about you, but the last time such invasive rules were placed on one particular group over another it took a Presidential Proclamation to abolish these threats to liberty. But we don't exactly need that to remedy this concern.

Re-educating Imperfect fleas: Day 3

Today is the day to break-in that new chalkboard and magical piece of chalk. By now your son's interest has been peaked as well as yours to drive out that low self-esteem. For the first time in his life, we will let his natural, instead of programmed talents out of his subconscious. On this day you both will decide if he goes toward the future or sideways towards stagnation. Remember to keep this initial training as light-hearted as possible. Don't seek to make any grandiose statements with his education at this point. Besides, he will take care of that himself if you let him lead.

Most parents are shocked at this third day of development when following this course. Keep in mind that a child's attention span is about three to five minutes based upon his calendar age. So be reasonable as well as responsible for your expectations. Don't let him lose a lifetime of interest by being frustrated by a routine that you would need a coffee break or a glass of wine to complete yourself. Also, keep in mind that if as a parent you had an education barrier routine that you shared in the past he could try to slip back into this routine. But the routine of one can easily be repeated while the routine of two can easily be broken. In short, relax and let him come down off of his sugar high before you move on.

At this point, you will not have to teach one single new thing. The only ground you have to cover as his dad is whatever he has already rehearsed in school. You want to show him that he can succeed where he might have failed in the past. Make him calm before he gets the chalk in his hand. Take the first problem that he received a failing grade for and tackle this one. If you can conquer just one problem the remaining issues in this same line of understanding will fall like dominos thereby allowing him to move onto the next level.

Go over the problem no matter how tough with him and simplify it to a level that you could understand it when you were two years younger than his calendar age. At this point forward you cannot touch the chalk or board except to erase it for him. You will be using the same type of writing paper he uses in school to explain the solution to the original problem just as his school teacher would. Explain to him how the magic of the chalkboard is only to be used for the talents that he was expressly born with.

Now that you and he are ready to let him write and then solve his first problem on the board. If he gets it right the first time you can respond the way his teacher would so he has continuity when he goes to school the next day. If she is a person that claps once he has achieved something do that. But if his teacher is a person that does not because it would appear as favoritism then do not do this. If he gets the problem, he placed on the board wrong then don't overreact.

The biggest problem in training or should I say leading people to their higher good is that we change our attitude based upon the rightness or wrongness of the problem solved.

In the real world if he gets something wrong, he will need to be reinforced just as I show you here. He will have to downshift for the correction and then move on in high gear to the solution. If he learns a pattern of you grimacing when he is wrong and clapping when he does right, he is being misled by you. Later on, in life your responses will serve as condemning emotion as he finds hi place in the world. As I say initially try to limit the time with the magic chalkboard to under an hour. If he ever in vibes the drive to push on without you then let that time be extended until he shows frustration or a willingness to play.

Since this piece of chalk and board were placed here to be used for him to grow into his own individual version of Einstein it should not be used for either play or frustration. I think it best that you get a smaller hand-held chalkboard and a small piece of chalk for play. You will find that his play board will become a place where he continues to solve the problems of life. The second thing you will prepare for this the third day of training is to nurture whatever career he desires to build. Allow for him the information he needs for his dream to become a reality. What you are looking to do is incorporate library grade skilled books in that trade that replicate his current skill level.

This type is much easier to gravitate to than the current system we use to train children. In this upcoming section, I am going to explain how you got to the level of needing to train at home this way. I want you to know why boys are becoming class-clowns in record numbers over their female counterparts. This information has nothing to do with left or right brain activity or reasoning. It has nothing to do with the myth that all boys fidget in their class-room chairs

The chief issue trying to end this crisis of confidence in the boy is not in taking on an array of feminine traits to pass through the twelfth grade. The key to his emotional development and well-being in school or out is to allow him to be the boy he was born to be as opposed to what makes society feel comfortable in his presence. Ask most any man who was raised prior to the new indoctrinations of male and they will tell you that they enjoyed their childhood. The truth is, no matter what time in history, the male has never been expected to complain about what he has been put through or grown through.

Take a snapshot of the average adult male's memory to see what childhood traits they share in common. Most men reminiscing about good times with cherished friends remember the days they walked into a classroom with an absentee teacher; only to come face to face with, a substitute teacher of the day. If these men once boys were slackers in school or their homework were not up-to-par they would be glad to see this unwelcomed substitute indeed. In these classrooms, most of the children usually feel a sense of relief, especially if the teacher that had been replaced for the day was a tyrant. This goes doubly true if that absentee teacher saw you as a kid with no possibilities for the future. But even if they were not in your best interest, you still had your parent's; or did you?

The parent will usually fail the child before the child fails the parent.

It is bad enough if a teacher that we cherished acknowledgement by felt this way about us, but what if it came from your parents at the same time? What if they too believed that you would amount to less than nothing as an adult? Would you have an incentive to rise above their expectations for you? In the United States, and around the world, we have a tendency to blame only the teacher for the failures of the student but what of the parent-teacher. I tell you that most children have failed their way out of life long before they had learned to stand-up at the side rails of their baby crib.

What we as adults don't take into account are that the longest running school our children ever attended was that of the home they were born. Imagine if you will that you have spent upwards of eighteen years with the same teacher in a one-room school-house called home. It was a well-meaning, mother or father that made the difference to whether we became inspired by life or demotivated through it. If we grew up in a home to where it seemed like our parent's phoned-in care-giving then you have, what I refer to as a substitute parent.

As substitute parent we act in the same spirit of a babysitter, as if they were waiting for the child's real parents to come and pick them up. This parent, although meaning no harm, remained mainly involved with their career personal life or free space more than with a child. In other homes, the parent could seemingly try to do their best by the child, but the word "best" does not pass muster in the eyes of even the parent who utters this truth in a supportive setting.

Shoot, the statement, "my parents did the best they could" would be a joke in any other industry. Would you call a national pizza chain on your cell phone and have them send "the best they could pizza?" Would you allow a surgeon to operate on you who got through medical school, "healing people the best he could?" no, you would want the people on both sides of your coin to give service beyond measure.

As great, or as less we believed our own upbringing to be, understand that you were challenged, and changed by that experiment. I refer to this altering of the individual spirit we were born to be as, switched at birth. You see most everyone breathing was never meant to be the image they project morning. In truth, if you were not born to those same parent's; but born instead twenty-two blocks south; you would be a very different person today. I can tell you for a fact that your thoughts and opinions about life, politics and wealth would be completely different from the belief you carry today.

Why is this? It is mainly because you were completely altered by the experiences that your parents went through in their childhood, overlapping onto your uniqueness. In effect, your parent's without knowing were preparing you for their past more than for your dreams and goals of the future. In changing our children from their original intention, we miss out on producing persons who could come up with cures for a disease, new inventions, and peace in the midst of a global-warming planet. To find out what you could have, or should have been by now; we have to venture back into your innocence of childhood. We will return to your child in a minute but I want you to know where your thought processes came from before you attempt to pass them on.

One day your child, like yourself will ask, who am I, and why am I here? We ask ourselves this puzzlement because sooner or later we realize that something was stolen from us that would make our life's journey a little bit smoother and easier. Without our permission, we have been modified from our original birth design which leaves us with a feeling of emptiness and loneliness wherein we never find satisfaction unless our course is corrected. This book was written to assist you, not with blame for your parent's. It was meant to yield to you that course correction and put you back on track for your child's life's mission.

Let me first start out by reminding you that you are very much a unique individual. There was no one ever born like you and after you die there will be no repeat of your exact DNA sequence in this entire universe. When you look into the dark of space of the night sky at the stars pondering the vastness of space; understand that you make up part of that vastness. To this date, I have never recalled meeting one new Imperfect boy who was ever the clone of any previously born person. What I have witnessed is that by the time that same baby has arrived towards adulthood he has been altered by parents and society to that experience.

Gone from his energies is that once lovable baby boy who once cooed back from the side rails of his initial baby carriage. Replaced by that memory is an overlay of how he should react based upon his parent's and neighbors' desires; buttressed against our race, gender, and income bracket. The very same income level he aspires to is the same he will one day seek the shelter of retirement from. But we are more than these simple task and summations. I tell you that boys were never placed here as mere servants to a governmental system of education or women. Most individuals that have ever sat in on one of my seminars or listened to one of my radio shows were merely seeking one thing. They were desperately soul searching the unique individual, "self" they lost during infancy. I can tell you now, as I told them then, that this journey without careful consideration, guidance, and inspiration can be one of the lowliest journeys you could ever take if you are seeking to find yourself through MGTOW. This is why it is important to assist your child in the great equivocation of past resentment for unaccomplished goals.

How large is the problem of lost identity in the world of men, once children? Currently, there are three-hundred-sixty thousand births each day worldwide of totally separate and distinct individuals; and approximately half of those births are male. But, before the sun has set on those "XY" chromosome births the next afternoon, plans must be made to convert these males into part of the wider collective. I am not referring to, "The Collective" as associated with, "The Borg" in the Star Trek series; although this comes pretty close to what all new arrivals of the species human face through parenting and environment training.

I am speaking to that certain push, and pull that is required in order to raise a child; as much as the struggle for the child to whom that undesired rising is being thrust down upon. But one thing that remains underestimated by both is that they will forever be locked, co-creators of their future selves. While a father scratches his head, desperately pondering why his pre-teen son is creating a trash dump out of his bedroom; he forgets his own past rebellions. He willfully chooses to overlook that his progeny is merely mimicking something that either he once possessed or self-righteously refuses to address in order to bait him son towards a sense of piety. The well-intentioned father is left to wonder, where in the hell, did I go wrong in raising this boy.

In this progeny puzzlement rest all of the answer to most of life, and the unrest in almost every home with families. What we as parent's fail to acknowledge is that we are only responsible for assisting our children in their arrival towards adulthood. It is not our jobs to reinvent that individual's persona into our youthful selves. As parent's, we mistakenly get frustrated when our individually crafted little ones do not turn out to be just like the dusty mold we built for our past dreams, and goals. Even worse still are the parents who get absolutely frustrated when they find out their child chooses to follow too closely their life-path in which they wished themselves to be free.

Re-educating Imperfect fleas: Day 4

"Knowing Why Your Son became Who HE Is"

*"Most adults are striving to fix the flaws given them
by their parent's, while gainfully imposing those same
challenges and limitations on their children's personal freedoms."*

Charles Rivers

Switching Story #1 Calming down the motivated child: By the time you were able to pull yourself up at your own crib-side; your parents had differing ideas about altering your future. Did they do these things out of spite or malice? No, but for the change that became you, it might as well have been. Let's imagine for a minute that you were born a very excited and boisterous baby. But you have no idea of that past because you only see yourself as you are in the mirror as an adult. In these motivated childhood behaviors, your parent's feared that you would not be accepted down the road in school and in life. They imagined that with this trait you could not make it financially in the future; due to the fact, that society has a place for overly-excited adult males.

Overly-excited men, in your parent's estimation, never made it to the top of the fortune 500 companies. In their reality, overly-excited men were those adults who got into a lot of public fights and ended up getting arrested frequently. Overly-excited boys entering pre-school were those kids who got sent home with a bunch of notes for inability to control their own behaviors. Knowing these self-imagined facts your parents formulated a grooming package for you that would allow them plenty of time to convert you to a more subdued yet manageable boy or girl entering pre-school.

What they did not understand then was that if you cage a freed spirit, it will rebel, and ultimately even against its own individual design. To confirm your behaviors to the impeccable child in a fictitious perfect society; they acted to control your individualism on your behalf. Every time they witnessed you being too excited, they either sat you down or drew you closer to their person. In public, while walking down the street; they grasp your hand to prevent you from venturing off too far on your own. When these measures did not take a hold, they began to punish you, after you reached the age in which things that mattered could be withheld from your pleasure.

They purchased or checked out volumes of books that explained how withholding sugar from hypersensitive-children would calm their spirits down. But they never had you diagnosed with this condition. Because of the learnings towards over-excitement, they began to substitute those sweet-toothed coveted cravings in your diet for healthier treats. By the time you were able to be admitted to that preschool learning, they had designed the perfect Franken-Child. They had inadvertently changed you forever from the light of this world person you were born to be to a new matrix of the perfect student. They now had a shell of a son who had his spirit snatched from him in order to be groomed toward a better future salary.

They had a child that would sit down, and do what anyone and everyone in authority wanted he or she to do at will. In you, they had someone who fearfully went through life as adults do, far too early in life; do to that molding process. You learned to dance to the music they did; to laugh at the television shows they enjoyed. Because of their grooming, you began to enjoy the privileges of a disciplined life. The abilities and talents you were born with that can only free-flow from an undeterred child, began to flow from you no longer.

Since you behaved far differently than the other children in your age category, you were given more leadership responsibilities early on. You were virtually forced to sign up for advanced positions of study as your teachers believed you could handle these because of your outward manageable behaviors. There were times when you felt lost in your desperate attempt to just keep up with the demands of being too disciplined a young adult; too early on in life. Because of this altered upbringing, you found out like most children remade-over this way. You found out that you faced very scary cross-roads once you grew closer to graduating high school.

You questioned, do I progress on to college in an attempt to satisfy my parent's desires or do I drop out because I need some time to find myself?

A few years down that same confused road and you found yourself with an addiction to temporarily soften the pains of not living the free-spirited life you would have designed for yourself. In some cases, you grew to be stuck with a current reality that mirrors your nightmares more than it does your dreams. Worse still you find that you are now married with children of your own and raising these little ones with the same antiquated ideas that your parents tried to pass onto you.

"Laughter, in the wrong context is more damaging than any weapon. For laughter against a tender heart prompts a soul to reject everything that makes it an individual"

Charles Rivers

Switching Story #2 Speeding up the subdued child: Let us look at that same story in the reverse teachings. For if someone can be raised to be mellowed against their own will than someone can also be groomed to be motivated beyond their farthest wishes. Starting from the delivery room, as your parents held you in a warm blanket; they noticed that you were not in their estimation a motivated child. In fact, in their worried eyes, you seemed a little listless and out-of-it.

At this moment they came together in a twisted agreement that you needed to be motivated in order to be successful in some far-off distant future. Remember, they meant you no harm in changing your behaviors beyond the fact, that they wanted you to be accepted by a faster society. In effect, they wanted you to be able to blend in, and not be laughed at for who you were naturally born to be.

The largest danger to this blending process is that you become a monotone individual. There is no greatness that comes forth from a group of like-minded followers minus you as lead. Those newly minted parents of yours mentally visualized the students many years before you could even begin to gum solid foods laughing at you.

They cringed at the idea of your fellow students deriving pleasure from teasing you incessantly over your lazy-eye. In this, they could not honestly live with themselves if you faced one minute of hurt. So, it was agreed that since you had a look that appeared to society to be slothful, they would work to blur that issue your person. Since you were not really expected to enter formal school for another five years, they figured they had plenty of time to alter your psyche. From that day forward, it was agreed that you would have to be sped up. After all, no child could expect to get a successful career if they appeared to be or were actually too slow to understand what was taught in college.

In their narrow-minded belief given to them by society; the slowest boys were predominantly poorer on the other side of town. Weren't the school systems on that side of town too rough a place for him to raise their grandchildren? Wasn't it the slower boys who were more aggressive, and picked fights with the more astute children all around them? Finally, wasn't it those slower boys who ruined the family tree with their offspring four generations beyond their parent's death? Sure, all these things sound funny enough for a child who has just been placed in his first pair of diapers but that is how it all starts.

Long before you were able to spill that first milk-filled sippy cup on your high chair your parents had begun to redesign you mentally in order brace you against a perceived world that they felt did not kindly accept them. As you progressed in school your parents enrolled you in every sporting event, they could find in order to give you a competitive edge. They placed you in as many motivating activities to force a perceived slothful attitude out of your being as if it were an infection; and not the person you were born to be. From this upbringing, you could have turned out in a myriad of fashions that I can't even begin to name here but you survived it.

In other homes, you have upbringings where the parent's believed that they were not as smart as their own son in his youth and wanted them to exceed beyond their wildest dreams. But in this profession, it is only marginally better than the parent's worst nightmares and cuts far too short the child's ultimate dreams and fantasies. There are homes where the male is not as naturally gifted as the parents in education. In this abode, the parent's if out of touch with their own humanity never ends up accepting his uniqueness over his perceived deficiency as a slight towards them.

In the over two decades of teaching, I do not believe, that I have ever met any adult who had ever struggled with an adult issue. Most adults, be they rich or poor always had a childhood issue plaguing their current free-will decisions. They could easily recant to me without fail, something that their parent(s) did to either make their past or their present a living hell. This story held the same, no matter whether the parent(s) were religious, agnostic, wealthy, or lived in stark poverty. In order to address my seminar participant's unmet dreams and goals, I knew I had to first address who or what it was they thought they truly were.

My first challenge over two decades ago was a young man named Martinez. Martinez on the initial meet explained to me how he had been adopted as a child to a family of modest means on the Latino side of town. Although Martinez was a Caucasian male, he was proud of his dual-upbringing but he had self-esteem issues.

He admitted to me in less than fifteen minutes of knowing me that he always thought that he was nothing. Upon hearing this, I grabbed both of my knees and bent over laughing right in front of him. I retained my composure as I began to see him tear-up at the sight of me laughing. He said are you laughing because I am nothing or trying to make fun of me. I placed my hand on his soldier and I said something that I would recommend you use to the student you are trying to motivate.

I said, Martinez, I have never met anyone, and I do not mean anyone that was not worth a million dollars. I said and by the time we finish with building up your esteem, you will know this also. Because of the family that Martinez grew up in the company they believed that no one could make it in a competitive environment without accepting low for themselves and low positions to survive. But I was not into survival just for the sake of surviving or anyone around me doing the same.

In your daily push to motivating underperforming little ones that come from this type of mindset, you are going to have to push them out of that mindset long before you can push them out of a negative environment. I am happy to say that Mr. Martinez was one of my greatest success stories and that nothing but success will follow him, his newborn child and his career successes throughout the remainder of his life.

Like Martinez, most MGTOW men will eventually feel a longing for what their life could have been. Ultimately every young man will taste the emptiness that only comes with unmet desires. The human mind can't begin to fathom how wide and deep unmet dreams mean to our souls. Because of the decoupling, you went through in child-hood altered your life's mission from your original design. Because you had nothing that was your desire to replace it you decided to join with the worlds plan for your life. That plan meant growing up, getting a job, marrying a woman who barely tolerates you and your children.

Those child-hood grooming techniques changed everything from choosing our friendships to our day of death. Some men grew bitter by this theft of life grew to hate their parent's like hell and love their friends like heaven. We became attracted closer to our friends believing them to be just as we with problems, challenges, and equal rebellions. But what if your most trusting friend is not their true selves also and you are in actuality being drawn to a false positive?

Holding our parent's accountable for a life we can change in an instant is equivalent to crying over a glass of spilled milk while being the owner of a dairy farm. As you move onto the next section, let us venture towards a brighter future by understanding and unraveling our made-up past. I believe that if you are dissatisfied with your current life, it means that you are not living your gifts. Maybe you are merely living out the expectations of everyone around you except the person within you. In knowing this, you have found your cause to change.

Re-educating Imperfect fleas: Day 5

"For the parent declares, "this child is nothing like me!" The child responds boldly and smartly, "Thank God!"

Charles Rivers

"Knowing Which Parts of You to Undo"

The question of, who is I, has always been asked and will be as long as people raise boys to men. But let's find out who you were prior to that past tense upbringing called normal. Since you did not choose the home you were born to, or the school's you attended it is a safe bet that the fix was in long before you got the idea to search for the "you" within your person. Typically, in my experience, if you are a fast-paced person who desires to be a more relaxed individual then these are leanings towards your original design. On the other hand, if you are a calmer person with a never-ending desire to scream out and increase your energy, than this may be your original design.

Now it may not be that easy to diagnose everyone in these two veins, but for many of us, we have but two or three steps to recovering our individuality. It took the person you get dressed in front of the mirror, eight changes to arrive at what you mentally visualize. Now keep in mind, I did not say what you physically see but mentally see. Understand that when you were first born you had not as yet become self-aware. The first step in your birth was that the universe invited you to your mother's womb as you were and without the aid or assistance of any outside correction, transformations or influencers.

The first change that occurred to your person was that your parents sought to reinvent you into the mold of your immediate family's desires for a child with your gender. The second change, your parents visited upon your person was to make you acceptable to your extended family members. The third change was your parent's engineering the plans to make you acceptable for your race and culture. The fourth change, your parents tried to instill upon you was by preparing you for the mold of the perfect formal educated child. The fifth change, your parents began to develop in you was your religion or lack of it for your home. The sixth change was in making you a socially acceptable human being into the society of your birth country.

The seventh change, you were instructed on who or what was the enemy or threat to your existence, based on your parent's beliefs and the local news. The eighth and final change, other less important doctrines like the introduction to, Santa Clause, your immediate homes income standards and the like were continually trained to you. All of these doctrines were constantly reinforced in order to give you an identity that would not be taken away with the introduction to public schooling or your closest friends. Yes, you would not be allowed to have a broader mindset at that age because your parents had not developed one over their entire lifetime enough to give you.

I am not meaning to come down hard on your parent's, as these ideas of raising you are the only ideas beyond books that they had to go on up till that time. Under their tutelage, unless they grew up, learning how to be themselves, how could they teach you to be anything different? Under their grooming, how could you teach your baby to be any different? Even a great parent who raises their child to be themselves ends up bracing their progeny against the laughter of a world that would prefer them to be nothing more than a clone of the local community's backdrop.

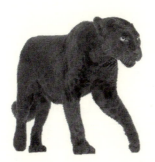

Panther Feminist
(The Sell Out)

"Just as deadly to female as she is to male, the elusive Panther Feminist has willingly sold more women into career-bondage than any plantation owner that has ever existed."

Charles Rivers

    She was the architect and pioneer of the myth of equality of sexes. She sits on her thrown from up high, not as a worker but as a ruler above the women's backs that she is allowed to sacrifice in her zeal to take down males of any society. She is the queen of double standards in her trickery to never be held at fault for the destruction she leaves in her wake. If she were not a female, the world would see for themselves just how militaristic her war game was against humanity. If you google any of the top feminist incomes, homes or cars you will find one of the largest disparities of wealth. Not the disparity of man to woman, but woman to woman. For the Panther Feminist knows only wealth through using the everyday woman's struggles to enrich her pocket-book. Over the entire chapter we are going to look at things, such as the myth of equality and how it has affected your home and the pockets of the women in charge of this charade.

Forewarning: You are going to see me refer to the modern-day Radical Feminism Movement as a movement to enslave men. You will see me refer to slavery, Hitler and other dominating forms in history. But I want you to understand that I am not blaming my white MGTOW brothers and that this is merely a history reference. What I will be offering is that same brother the knowledge he needs to go directly, toe-to-toe with the woman who would blame him for those events in history.

I have to approach this subject in the most candid way I can in order to give you the red pill you need to wake up and stop being a cog of society. In this chapter you will definitely go deeper into the rabbit-hole and find out what was always done in plain sight of your sleeping eyes. You will more than likely need to rest one whole day after reading this section to take it all in. And if you go to work the next day, I guarantee you will not see the world as you did the day before now. Remember, the Women's Liberation Movement sought to change males by altering the makeup of little boys. So it is that this awakening will start once again with the damage to you as a boy before you became man. Are you ready to take the red pill? Remember, you could take the blue pill and go back to the uncomfortable, comfortable life you had been living.

Taking the Red Pill

It is now more detrimental for a human baby boy to be raised in the home of his birth mother than any other setting; if his psyche and sense of self-worth are to remain intact. An entire generation of boys has been raised up to do only what makes them feel happy and good on the inside. This trick was done purposely to feminize them away from past test of endurance that made them great. This Radicalized Feminist rearrangement doctrine has led to the first generation of the most damaged young men the planet has ever witnessed. This generation of feminist rearranged boy's greatest desire in life was to play video games all day long while doing drugs with their pants halfway down his ass. Now sure enough they did this in a defiant movement towards a past that they felt was unjust but the biggest injustice was done to their future and she relished this with open arms.

If she could just take away the pride that men had to be themselves by taking the father out of the home her purpose would be served. The religion of masculinizing girls and feminizing boys had materialized a culture of young men who were lost to themselves and angered by the experience. It produced boys that would go into occupied schools and public places and mow-down everyone in sight with automatic weapons. Yes, female's liberation in its attempt to broaden rights for girls ended up giving fatherless boy's too many open ended possibilities that ultimately drove them headlong into the Unemployment Zone.

But look what came of this pseudo-science experiment, how did those boy's that were bred to enjoy the foolishness of youth fair? Did being free from fathers and all responsibility make today's average grown man happy? Nope, this is one of the first generations of men ever been born that are completely miserable with the freedoms of a non-accountability fatherless home brought with it. And what of the flip-side of the gender equation, how had his female counterpart faired? Well, if everyone hadn't noticed by now, the last generation of females raised under a liberation theology has done quite excellent for themselves with the help of mom and the Federal Government.

Little girls have been encouraged to seek out, and take responsibility wherever they may have found it. They have stood firm shouldered against every test that has come against them over the last forty-plus years. They have amassed wealth, in the form of investments, mansions, and yachts in some cases. Some women within the one percentile of feminist have gone even further to owning corporations and private jets. But how did those better-fairing ladies feel on the scale of personal satisfaction? Among women, historical poled statistically reported that they felt themselves to be the most miserable generation of women that ever came to be. They are not personally fulfilled as much as their bank accounts are financially fulfilling. The generation of Radical Feminization had hit a snag in its untested science of switching roles. In the estimation of the political scientist, it was in danger of heading for a backlash by its own members. It was definitely the inspiration for the MGTOW movement back to sanity for men. Lastly its spawned defeat for its own presidential nominee, Mrs. Hillary Rodham Clinton at the hands of the very same men her movement had sought to marginalize.

In the first generational challenge of placing a woman as president would be feminisms hallmark failure. There would be many reasons bantered about as to why the first woman to get the presidential nod failed twice to place first in that most hotly contested contest. Instead of her admitting that, yes, we had made mistakes along the way and that we needed to improve ourselves in order to regain our member's confidence she didn't. She didn't admit it to us and certainly not herself. In fact, for her second attempt at breaking the glass ceiling, she dusted off her same tired act and list of donors. Unfortunately showing up to face Mr. Trump proved easier than being trumped by him.

A second defeat within the same century for such a coveted milestone would prove the last grab for power for the movement. And as a writer to the truth I can tell you that I am very much pleased with the outcome. I do not tout either party as a solution for what ails this country but I know feminism as a religion is a cure for nothing. In her loosing Mrs. Clinton also leaves a legacy behind in that she dodges responsibility in a job that would have required responsibility over a twenty-four-hour day. Mrs. Clinton could not admit defeat on the night of the election nor in her subsequent book, "What Happened." Jokingly, I think the book would have been better named, "What Had Happened Was." But if Mrs. Clinton could not admit defeat to herself, Feminist or the international media than who are we left to blame for this public trouncing?

Does anyone of us finally have the balls to say that the only reason Mrs. Hillary Clinton lost the young men's vote in two key presidential nominations was that males no longer trusted women? Oh, I don't mean that they don't trust women because they don't have a pair of balls. I mean they don't believe that any female has a male's best interest at heart; period. For the good or progress that

Radical Feminism brought to the lives of girls and women, it brought only hell and criticism to the lives of their sons.

It had apartheid fathers from sons and men from women as callously as a slave master would scatter an enslaved mother's baby from her desperately clinging arms. Those fatherless anguished boys grew one day into avenging men and those men into a surprising new Underground-Railroad voting bloc. Women's Lib had unknowingly placed the last nail in its own coffin by birthing the opposite of its aims in turning boys against the movement. None of us can really be surprised because history has always shown us this outcome.

Usually when the powers-that-be are in charge they brush away the concerns of the marginalized people that are not like themselves and in this case, they were male. Mrs. Clinton had erroneously judged grown men as sexist pigs, not willing to vote for her but she missed the obvious evidence landed by that key voting group in two elections. In Mrs. Clinton's first election there was a large contingent of eighteen-year-old males that were just ten years old at the mid-point of Feminist Movement. During her second election, she faced a new group of young boys that were only ten years of age during the waning years of the Feminist Movement. The movement for all intents and purposes had its greatest motivations behind it. In fact, in my estimation, it had lived a much longer life than the short run Black Power Movement that sputtered in the late 1970s.

Try as you might, no one could fault a failed popularity contest for president on sexism in a country replete with a generation of men and women who had been raised by feminist. The largest group of voting age men and women during Secretary Clinton's first and last election campaigns were well versed and respective of the tenants of feminism and the "ERA Bill." The ERA Bill or Equal Rights Amendment as reintroduced by U.S. Representative Martha Griffiths (D-Michigan) in 1971.

Sure, I admit it was a long-shot to even try and beat the novelty of the first black president in Mr. Barack Obama after his 2007 presidential campaign primary begun. But what happened in the next election?

Why did the so-called, "Old White Guy's Generation" take the presidency with relative ease? This was the first generation that pollsters knew that a woman would be a shoo-in for the presidency. With the most popular president since Abraham Lincoln in the form of Barack Obama out of the picture, there was no way they expected her to fail. Since Mr. Obama claimed a landslide majority of the black vote, they assumed she would claim the equivalent in the female vote. And with men being washed-up with the self-hating doctrines of the Feminist Movement surely, they would give her a free pass into history. They thought, why would a country that professes to fight for the liberties of foreign countries with precious U.S. soldiers blood turn down its chance to make things right at home?

I'll tell you what happened. For the first generation in U.S. history women dominated every form of discipline in a little boy's life born between 1966 and the late 1990s. She was his mother in a struggling single-parent home. She was his daycare teacher when his mom could not make it home on time. She was his babysitter when his mom had to work late night.

She was the school-bus-driver who angrily made him take his seat on the way to school. She was his school teacher who sent him begrudgingly for defending himself straight to the principal's office. She was the heartless principal when he arrived at that office who expelled him immediately to that empty motherless home. She was his local police officer who watched him from a patrol car awaiting him to do something wrong so she could arrest him.

She was the judge in whose estimation he was unjustly sentenced for a longer term than his female counterpart for the same crime. She was his wife who gave him hell every day, despite how well he tried to provide for her and his children. She was his boss, who held executive positions even on the career he chose as his dream job. These boys, now young and middle-aged men were tired of her and her domineering condescending attitude and they were ready for their own revolution.

These boys, now voters didn't ever get the chance to see what equality was in a liberated America but they damn sure knew what it wasn't.

They had sisters they could not win a race against because their mothers cried out, "let your sister win!" So, this male voting bloc had nothing in their youth to prove to them the myth of gender equality. There was nothing in the boy's preteen years that would indicate a society assisting both boys and girls as equals to get ahead. The only thing boys noticed was a rehashed version of his mom's voice during that same sidewalk race. As teens, boys witnessed nothing that assured him society would shuffle the deck fairly in both of their favors. In his enlistment within his chosen branch of the U.S. Military, he still marveled how the rules were twisted to allow his female counterpart to appear just as equal.

He knew full well that on one hand the government called females equal to males while still only having intentions to draft men in the next war. In his mind, since there was nothing from birth to voting age that resembled the equality cry of the Radical Feminist, he decided to change his mental vote. Maybe those older men when I was a boy were right when they said the government was fixing the system like a player who throws a basketball game for money. Like previous generations of American citizens these boys were ready for voter insurgency motivated by the disapproval of fat cats at the end of each generational cycle.

Even in this generation young teenage boys have formed their own version of the MGTOW Movement known as TGTOW. TGTOW or (Teens Going Their Own Way) has had enough of watching men get screwed by women. They refuse to stand in line and wait their turn to be the servants we were. This movement was born in the country of Australia but will soon spread world-wide. You would have expected this movement to have taken root in the States first with the ass-whooping young male voters gave to the former First Lady. You would have expected boys here who were tired of not being able to swing a cat without hitting a woman to drive this issue home. Boy, little do most mothers know that they are now birthing the death of their own cherished movement.

The modern feminist mother in her son's eyes had come to represent little more than an edict issuing patriarchal figure like Robert Young, the male role model on the 1954 television show, "Father Knows Best." With every year that went by his once protective mom who intervened to saved his hide from father's raft became, "Single Mom, the Disciplinarian." She was now, not only his mother, but by default, his father. It was her genders face these young boys had to come to despise when they did something wrong and not that of a male.

It was she who had allowed his school system to administer a lethal addictive drug to him in the form of Ritalin. In this drug, the Radical Feminist found a very neat and tidy ally never before in their arsenal of tricks. No longer did they have to try to elicit the U.S. Governments help in the pansification of infant boys but they had a drug that would do it with self-administering. In this drug, the drive that males had naturally exhibited in the over two-hundred years of this country's history had all but been vanquished. Now, the girls who could not compete with boys in the past had a new reason to hope.

I don't really believe without the addition of Ritalin to millions of boys along with the belief of inferiority girls would have progressed so far. Now society sees that if you want equality you don't have to rise to the level of competing with boys. No, all you have to do is lower boys to the level of female enthusiasm and you can walk all over them. According to the United Nations, the U.S. produces and consumes about 85 percent of the world's methylphenidate.

In school, unlike at home when he raced his sister down the sidewalk, he didn't have to hear his mother's voice saying, "Let your sister win!" The new motto for this campaign became better aptly named, "If you can't beat them, drug them." Gone were the initial fail-safes of previous generation where mommy played good cop while dad the bad cop. It would have been too easy to say all these voting males were sexist if each and every male agreed with one another. But unlike women, males have no because that unites such loyalty except for women's angry behaviors towards the male species. Plain and simple little boys got tired of being made a scapegoat for something that Christopher Columbus and crew decided to do at the last ball before the big sail. There was no one who was left not indoctrinated by a feminist attitude to block victory for the first female feminist president. So how then could we blame a no-contest vote on an entire generation of boys raised by a modern-day feminist?

Wouldn't anyone believe just as Hillary that it should have been a cake-walk on greased ice? Well, let me clue you in on one little secret. Men are not women and they are not beholden to anything but good leadership when it comes to an election. Having a penis is not a literacy test or a poll tax that a candidate has to have in order to run for the highest office of the land.

Although those boys, now men were raised by mothers they were never truly beholden to a feminine way of life. Try as you might you will never be successful at getting a generation of men to love women who hates them with a passion. Try as you might the boys on the local level can see the women who act afraid of him when he walks down the street. The males on a local level know that the woman staring at them out of the window just called the cops on him for doing absolutely nothing.

Try as you might men on the local level who vote on a national level cannot be fooled with or without the red pill. We know full well that it is females on a local level that act like tyrants on the job. We know that it is women who are responsible for making sure things go right in our lives that really could not care one iota just because we are men. Sure, you have women that are nothing likes this but those women don't stand up at any time when we are being mistreated. They don't stand up and come to the rescue as a man would if she was being attacked on the street, trapped in her car or stranded with a flat tire. In short, men got tired of an entire generation of women who wanted the same for men as the creature in the first movie, "Independence Day," for us to DIE.

There is that separation in a little boy's life that occurs around the age of six that won't allow him to see mom's one-sided point of view. Especially if that view comes with instructions that his way of life must perish in order to benefit the gender that despises him most. This growth period in a boy's life is the target of feminist who wants to make boys effeminate in an effort to dull their competitive edge. What young boys begin to see is that feminism hurts them the stronger it seeks to marginalize his freedoms.

What most mature aged voting males had come to see was that feminism no longer sought the rights of women but to maliciously take every right a man had. Long before the first electoral votes had been tallied, men and women alike from an entire generation of feminism were fed-up. Mothers who had decent sons cast their votes for sanity over a form of modern-day slavery for his future.

Modern Feminist for the first time lost by their actions the coveted vote their grandmothers had dreamed of in Mrs. Clinton. Mother's lost the respect of the men they had intentionally under-nurtured over the last fifty years as they built their precious careers. It mattered not the gender of the voter; just that feminist had begun to act worse than the men they had for so long derided as evil.

What those young boys, now men viewed, for the most part, was that women saw men as something either to use, abuse or to allow them to get over on. They felt marginalized, minimalized, put upon and like the Vietnam War Veterans, spat upon. As he grew into a young man, he remembered the older men saying, "Watch out for those women or they will take everything you got!"

In his youth he would have easily brushed aside this information aside as the crazy rantings of an old man. But what happened with each passing year of our maturity is that the old man's words began to ring true. Unbeknownst to most mothers is that all little boys have the inside track at the woman's enemies camp. As young males, we have reared at her feet a privy to all of her seductive, secretive phone calls and misgivings about males. We overheard your conversations about the males you plan to hurt, steal from or sleep with.

But if a woman on the street engages a man in conversation, she somehow believes that he knows nothing of women's nature or misgivings. Somehow there still exists the opinion that women have mystical secrets about them, which they most certainly do not. The average boy is raised by his grandmother, his mother, his sister, his niece, his aunt, and female babysitters. If there was any mystery left, it went straight out of the window in his youth.

The problem with feminist theology is that they believe a woman can raise a boy as well as they can raise a girl but this is far from the truth. No one would advocate tomorrow that every father could raise his daughter without the input of the feminine nature but this is what we do to our boys. It is almost as if women wanted grown men not to have influence over their own children. But in doing this you do not prevent him from growing into a man nor can you promote him to your way of thinking with this behavior. This idea spawned the young boy with his pants down, the kid that would kill his fellow students and so on. It seems that the hardest battle the feminist agenda will fight will be, how can we make males accept our deceptive bullshit and not rebel?

I can tell you as a son of a once single mother that all young boys start out as feminist or pro-female. In fact, males to our own detriment believe in women far more than we do men. This belief is primarily based upon the fact that we are taught that females are nicer than males. We are taught just like our young female counterpart that all things masculine is either scary or dangerous. Because of this teaching, men do not allow the average boy into the group called man. He is not allowed entry until he can stop his own self-hatred. That's right, I said self-hatred. Most women that have a dislike for men try everything in their power to either neuter their boys or teach them to hate everything about themselves. Is there any wonder why males fight each other more as the generations go by instead of less?

This trick of turning men against one another was not pioneered by feminist but perfected by them. This behavior is more of a model from the separationist White Supremacist histories of the Ku Klux Klan and the Old South. You would readily accept this doctrine from that period of time more than a group that claims themselves to be more loving, giving, and decent. Oh, there it is again, the same behaviors from women are those of hate-filled groups instead of love-filled persons. It seems almost as if most adult women believed that men were birthed by other men and then raised in the woods alongside bears. Not that we were actually reared at her feet as she bad mouthed the species of man to include our fathers. That we were there when she diminished the value of men and uplifted the same behaviors in women.

That the only men she paid homage to exist only on the covers of those untold number of romance novels she kept at her bed-side. Every time a trusted woman in the lineage of man has disdain for him, she creates another no vote for any election or position of authority in his eyes. Not voting for women have little to do with gender and more to do with attitude. Hell, even women don't trust women once they have witnessed what the modern-day Feminist Agenda has destroyed. As the field of potential nominees emerges to face the current president in the next election, I don't believe that a woman will be successful at getting elected. I believe this because the man on the street who has to either pull a lever or press a button cast his vote on a local level with national intentions.

He cannot cast his vote for her after he has taken into account the woman on his street block. When he takes into account the scars of his verbally and physically abusive mother. His sister who molested him as a child and belittled him just for being male. His wife who has hindered him in his quest to be an equal co-parent of his children. No, I would wager you any amount of money that women are not on the move forward for their angry militant views against men but backwards with extreme prejudice. Only this time that backward move won't be supported by an estranged family she never kept in contact with, pretentious friends, ex-husbands denied visitation rights, children she under-nurtured or a community she never spent a moment of time in.

Forget about what you think of men for a moment. Do you honestly believe that a president such as Donald J. Trump could have been handed the White House so easily if all of the voting aged women were pleased with Radical Feminism? This billionaire, now Commander and Chief had to capture a rather substantial swath of the Feminist vote in order to even place in that race. Remember, the population of males is represented as only half of the U.S. in total and all of those males are not voting aged. There were women on voting day that were absolutely pissed about the way their movement had been driven off of the rails. So even with Mr. Trumps supposed sexism and abrasive rantings he still won. Do you remember some of the feminist lines that they wanted to hang Mr. Trump out to dry over? I list for you just a few of the sixty-one negative comments listed on, "The Weeks" website.

On Carly Fiorina
"Look at that face. Would anybody vote for that? Can you imagine that, the face of our next president? I mean, she's a woman, and I'm not supposed to say bad things, but really, folks, come on. Are we serious?"

On Hillary Clinton
"If Hillary Clinton can't satisfy her husband, what makes her think she can satisfy America?"

"If she were a man, I don't think she'd get five percent of the vote."

"Such a nasty woman."

On Megyn Kelly
"She gets out and she starts asking me all sorts of ridiculous questions. You could see there was blood coming out of her eyes, blood coming out of her wherever."

"Bimbo."

On the #MeToo movement
"It is a very scary time for young men in America, where you can be guilty of something you may not be guilty of. ... Women are doing great."

"You've got to deny, deny, deny and push back on these women. If you admit to anything and any culpability, then you're dead. ... You've got to be strong. You've got to be aggressive. You've got to push back hard. You've got to deny anything that's said about you. **Never admit."** [Via Bob Woodward's Fear: Trump in the White

House]

"I moved on her actually. You know she was down on Palm Beach. I moved on her and I failed. I'll admit it. I did try and f-ck her. She was married."

On the women of The Apprentice
"All of the women on The Apprentice flirted with me — consciously or unconsciously. That's to be expected."

On whether he's had sex with a black woman: "Well, it depends on what your definition of black is."

On women, generally
"Women have one of the great acts of all time. The smart ones act very feminine and needy, but inside they are real killers. The person who came up with the expression 'the weaker sex' was either very naive or had to be kidding. I have seen women manipulate men with just a twitch of their eye — or perhaps another body part."

"There's nothing I love more than women, but they're really a lot different than portrayed. They are far worse than men, far more aggressive, and boy, can they be smart!"

"I think the only difference between me and the other candidates is that I'm more honest and my women are more beautiful."

"26,000 unreported sexual assaults in the military — only 238 convictions. What did these geniuses expect when they put men & women together?"

To a female reporter: "We could say, politically correct, that look doesn't matter, but the look obviously matters. Like you wouldn't have your job if you weren't beautiful."

With all these lines and many more that were known prior to the election didn't even seem to slow him down. And what of the women who were staunched Feminist from the 1970's? I spoke once with a retired feminist friend of mine who said to me, "Charles, I believe some of that stuff we did during the Movement wasn't right at all."

I told her that it was good that she came clean with the facts but I told her that her opinion to me behind closed doors did not count. It doesn't count because she is telling it to me as many women do, in secret or in private, instead of in public where the seeds of Gender Apartheid had been planted and nurtured. But this book is not a diatribe about how one woman lost the presidency, but how women in total are losing the respect of their male counterparts they birthed to brand new heights.

We may be living in a time period where a woman can profess in public that she does not need a man but we also know that to be a bold-face-lie. When a woman utters these lines, I don't listen. It doesn't matter what you say out of your mouth as much as what her body says to her around midnight when she is feeling horny. At midnight in secret is when women dress up for clubs to chase the men, they say they hate. Why? It is because women are at their daily peak stage of testosterone. Testosterone is both sexes enhancement chemical around midnight each night for her and about day-break for men. At these times a woman's female friends can't scratch the itch she has on the inside of her body or mound. Yes, the modern-day liberated woman has power, the kind of power that only comes with expendable income but money doesn't buy you man's love.

"Money doesn't buy you love" was a famous line that women enjoyed hurling at men when they were the only bread-winners. At the printing of this book, a well-to-do liberated woman could now afford to buy whatever her heart so desired. She could buy a mansion if she was so inclined. She could buy the finest cars, jewelry, and a vacation to wherever she dreamed. She could even buy her daughters way into the most prestigious Ivy-League colleges and some have done just that this year. But the only thing she could not afford to buy with all of those coveted liberated dollars in the world was the modern-day MGTOW man. Yes, as much as her male counterpart similarly appreciated the finer things in life, he doesn't like being bought by women to get them.

Radical Feminist, on the other hand, has had no problem in selling themselves out or the men they engage courtship with to get "mad-cheddar" or money. Yes, to get what she wants financially, even forty-five years after pushing the ERA Amendment women are still willing to sacrifice their men, children, and humanity on the altar of the almighty dollar.

With the simple nature difference between the two genders reveals to us this. The average women will covet everything a male suitor owns financially before deciding if she wants to get into a relationship with him. Most males, on the other hand, accept women's finances sight unseen. For all of you blue piller's out there who are saying she has to protect her investments; then why don't you feel this way in reverse? Does this make blue pill swallowers idiots, or suckers to women, yes? Most women would never accept a man without his ability to take care of himself and her financially. But at least the male focuses on the woman's body and not what's in her, Louis Vuitton handbag.

The average male may be a sap when he falls for a curvy woman's figure walking past him. He may fall into her well-laid trap which she set for his innate weaknesses but again at least I say he is falling for her person and not her pocketbook. When a woman falls for a man's money that has nothing to do with him physically. Money has no bearing on his consciousness or humanity which is exactly why women have paid dearly in bad relationships with men.

If a man chose a woman based on income as she does him, he would never have a mate. If he chose someone who made more than him this would thin the field out to a very smaller percentage. If within that field he was looking for someone who would have his best interest in mind financially the field would diminish even further. If finally, he chose a woman who would be his lifetime mate and cater to his every financial whim that number would drop to maybe one. If he expected her to cover him after she had died through insurance then there would be no one left on that list. But somehow these are all of the thing's women aspire in a good man, in a world of all things equal.

> *"If Tiger Woods chose women with the same passion that he applied to the game of golf he wouldn't have a problem."*
>
> One man's comments during the Master's Tournament 2019

In this society as well as around the world, the modern feminist on the street neither has to justify her actions as she has a media outlet to handle that for her. The Radical Feminist television spokeswoman is at the top of the food chain in the gender female. She can be considered the Pied-Piper. She alongside her paid for victim cohorts have been featured on daytime talk-shows for over the past generation of television. Her stories are always the same, men are inherently bad and women are born angelically good. From her televised bully pulpit, she issues edicts of behavior to the women she believes beneath her station in order for them to do her bidding. She is a televised fraud and a fake nice woman. When the dust settles from this entire affair, they will point their fingers at her for fifty years as the cause for global catastrophe.

She is a broader inclusive speaker by mouth, but an exclusive actor behind closed door planning sessions. For a time, she has had the ability to pull the wool over even men's eyes. But one-by-one they awoke to the damage that she was trying to bring their way in order to amass wealth for herself. She knew full well just as the early cigarette ads for women did, that if you use hate, you can sell any product to women. As long as that hate is male-focused you will increase your viewership and wealth status. The same manufacturers wouldn't dare use anything but uplifting notes of harmony when selling a product to a woman.

In the future, the largest downfall will come to the companies that pandered to women against men. Once women use all of their expendable cash and credit, I am sure that these manufacturers will turn their attention towards men. But this daytime talk-show host knew that for years. She learned the tricks of the trade and sold her own gender into credit servitude to suit her commercial sponsors for over twenty-five years. When she had enough and earned a billion dollars for herself, she retired.

Surprisingly she still pedals hate to her gender in order to stay culturally relevant. But with generation, "Z" coming to adulthood her days of influence are numbered. I am not proud of her but ashamed that she is an African American woman who comes from a lineage of slaves who knew nothing but being hated by their captors. My question is that after all of that history, why would you be the one eliciting hate that would bring ruin and pain in the lives of other humans? As a self-proclaimed Feminist, she uses phony speeches of inclusiveness, equality and compassion for women; as actually code words for domination, selfishness and a take no prisoner's attitude.

She uses the government to rein in the same freedoms of men she seeks to expand in women. The Radical Feminist is not a lady to trust for she has the blood and pain of servitude of her own sisters on her hands. I can remember one afternoon when I was working to complete a task I had been putting off for some time on my job. An acquaintance of mine named Dan decided he wanted to elicit my support in helping the Black Community come to his cause. What Dan really wanted was a person like me from the Black Community to be the gentle token minority on his money-making charity. This is what the Racist Radical Feminist found in the woman who peddled hatred on TV for twenty-five years.

I declined his offer immediately and had grown tired of his repeated haranguing on the subject. I certainly was not in the mood to hear it rehashed again that day. So, I asked Dan a question that would be sure to let the air out of his money-making scheme. I said Dan, being that you are a Caucasian male why don't you want to help your own community over mine? I asked why anyone would jump over their own community issues to point out the fragility of another. He said it was because the Black Community was underprivileged and needed his support. I could barely contain my laughter when I told Dan that he didn't know all Blacks and that when Black people had a problem they normally turn to their families and not outsiders.

Men Going Their Own Way

I said the actual damage he needed to fix was not that of the black community but his own community. Since he believed his community was well-off, he was confused to my line of reasoning. Now keep in mind, Dan was a very well to do man.

I told Dan, that, you have a problem with the female of your race who calls herself a feminist, abandoning you, and leaving you behind. Dan asked, how so? I said the modern-day Caucasian Female is a decedent of the First Settlers that landed in Plymouth Harbor in the year 1620. I said if we can agree on that, we can also agree that she has been alongside the Caucasian Male for over three hundred and eighty-two years of this country's history, through good and bad times. He said, OK, I can agree with that much. I then asked him then why did she abandon you? He said do you mean my wife who divorced me? I said no, I mean how can someone that the Caucasian male supported for almost four centuries walk away from supporting him back after liberation.

How could she say that time period meant nothing, I am leaving you for dead? How can she look at you as if you were the only one responsible for slavery and that she was there enjoying the privileges against her will? How can she turn to vilify you as a white man and yet share the same skin color? She was alongside you when the black race you purport to want to help were placed in chains against their will, she was there. She was there when the Congress of the United States told her that if she would not join forces with the black female, they would give her the right to vote.

In believing Congress, she dropped the black woman from her crafted legislation on equal rights in order to get the right to vote. That same congress reneged as usual on that support and instead only voted to give women a symbolic day known as Mother's Day. In that day they enjoyed laughter at her expense by placing it on Sunday so it would not enjoy any of the rights or privileges of any other holiday would. They placed that day on a weekend where it would not impede with commerce or employees' rights and privileges.

Dismayed but never forgotten the Caucasian women rested her fight on this issue until the Black Power Movement rounded off the generation for Civil Rights for Black Citizens. She thought it best to broach the subject again since the country was turning towards rights for its black citizens. That same Caucasian woman who professed her strong desire for equality chased down her once enslaved sister in the late 1970's for round two of deception.

She asked the black woman who had, at last, gained the right to vote despite the white woman's support, if she would join with her in an attempt to reintroduce the same Rights Bill, she sold her out on sixty years earlier in 1914. I told Dan if any woman had the right to be liberated it was the Black Woman. For the Black Woman had gone from shackled slave to servant, to low wage earner for generations as the Caucasian woman fussed over how she should clean her house better while she sat.

I told him that it was beyond me how the Black Female or any female of color could join forces with someone who wanted to see them live and die with a marginalized second-class life. Even till this day, black women make less than their white female counterparts. We do indeed have an equality problem in America. Not of opposite genders but of the same equal genders. Recently, the Institute for Women's Policy Research stated that white women make about 81.5 cents per dollar that a white man makes. But black women make .61 cents per dollar as compared with the white man. Maybe for the sake of equality you should compare, women to women instead of women to white men.

You can't spell libe**rat**ion without placing a Rat at its core

In the title of "Libe**rat**ion" itself, you have the biggest rouse ever committed to paper. How can a woman be freed from something if she will be required to trade her freedoms as a slave for it? The word, liberation has its roots in the French definition liberty or libertine. The average liberated woman had been sold a raw bill-of-goods by the feminist that herded her angered emotions.

The average wife was told that she should not have to cook for her husband as this was a chore for a servant. Today that same average woman has a job as a liberated front-line cook at a restaurant making meals for minimum wage for over **600** people per shift. Doesn't sound a bit like liberation to me. The head feminist told women that she should not have to clean for her husband. The same average woman is cleaning **thirteen** rooms a day in a major hotel for less than minimum wage. Doesn't sound a bit like liberation to me.

Women were told that they shouldn't have to wash clothes for their husbands. Those same women now work for your local laundromat or dry cleaners with the responsibility of cleaning **hundreds** of peoples clothing each day. Doesn't sound a bit like liberation to me. The average woman was told by the chief feminist who is now a very wealthy woman that she shouldn't have to spend all of her precious time raising her own children.

Now, who do you guess is babysitting upwards of **forty-five** children a day for minimum wage down the street on your block? Bingo, the very same woman that was promised massive freedoms by destroying her own home. Doesn't sound a bit like liberation to me. Wait, didn't I read this story somewhere about a snake, an apple and a Garden of Eden somewhere before. Yes, the modern-day Radical Feminist is little more than a slave-trader to the Middle Passage off the coast of Western Africa in the 16th century. I encourage every female reader of this book to check out the salaries of your top feminist. But let's go back a minute more to the excitement of liberation.

Yes, opportunities abounded for women who were too put-upon at home with their controlling husbands. I ask you further, who is **sweeping** the floor late Christmas Eve in that sky-scraper of a building in your town? Who is driving a city bus as a liberated woman picking up upwards of **5,000** passengers a day while griping if she has to drive her husband half a block? As a driver, she is managing a day through dealing with passengers that tell her to either, go to hell, throw things at her or give her mean glances. Could it possible that all of these women have the potential for more real violence over the perceived violence feminist touted at home?

To this date I can find no uplifting position women have inherited enough to say thank you to Feminist for liberating me. Men have been working for thousands of years outside of the home and they consider it a living hell and not to be referred to as liberated. You cannot fool the average male that a job or a career will make him happy or free him. You can't convince him of this because despite him having a job he still does not know liberation from his wife, children or responsibilities. He still owes her the same duties today as he did forty-five years ago, plus newly created one's society seeks to free his wife from.

If women wanted to know the sheer ecstasy of a hard day of social mind-numbing games all she had to do was to ask any of the minority group of women. In truth, I said it is the black woman who should have been freed in liberation to relax to the same couch that the Caucasian woman's desires denied her. But I digress about Dan before I get too far off the subject of government-engineered freedoms that are more invasive than the demonstrative edicts passed down on the Colonist by King George the III.

The only danger of this entire premise is that there has never been freedom from or in a governmentally induced system. All one has to do is look upon world history to see the damage that any government has created when trying to present a balance of one group's concerns over another. In a governmental view of legislated equality, you have an inequitable treatment of Native Americans as opposed to White Americans. Remember, these are facts and not a condemnation of a history long since passed. I will leave that up to the pundits who stoke hatred for past transgressions.

In a government instituted equality, you have a system legislated as, "Separate but Equal." In a governmental system of equality, you have very physically demanding child labor, before the Child-Labor Law Act of 1938. In a government legislated equality, you have the twisting of the Equal Rights Amendment that allows boys to languish in order to make them pay penance for a system his government instituted against his female counterpart and not him. Typically, in this country or any other for that matter, the persons that have the most to gain from governmental heavy hand protection least want to yield those coveted privileges.

The group under the government's version of equity attempts to suppress the thoughts, feelings, and actions of their perceived enemies in an attempt to gain benefit for themselves. In this case that would be the rights of girls and women over boys and men. I yield you the following examples. Slavery in the United States benefited the Caucasian Race far more than the Black Race, the German Government and its treatment of the Jews. The Germans benefitted far more than the Jews.

The Ba'athist Party treatment of the Sunni under the government of Saddam Hussein. I would wager you real Saudi riyal dollars that the Bath Party benefitted far more than the Sunni Tribes under the rule of Saddam Hussein. The government and the top Pied-Piper always benefit financially from the loudest voices in the crowd and shares in the spoils of that voice until they lose financial and public prominence.

I tell you, that Radical Feminist who aligned themselves with the government are doing real and not perceived damage to all of our young boys of all races. In their grasp for the glory of wealth, they are attempting to make little boys feel inferior to girls. This poison of the water and stealing of one's identity and dignity before they are able to tie their own shoes is a dangerous road to go down. If any history of the world tells us that none of this last for long. There has been no group to date that has simply rolled over and allowed for their complete domination and wealth to be stolen. Countries that have attempted to do this go through civil wars, coups and peaceful exchanges of illegally attained power.

In essence, we are asking boys to hold themselves back in the race of life and let their sister win. This unequal way to redistribute wealth can only lead to tragedy for everyone involved. The human boy is now becoming a second-class citizen in his own country to his female counterpart. Why is this harmful you might say? Because globally we have established behaviors and norms for both genders that benefitted in some fashion. But unlike his female counterpart if a young boy does not find a career, he cannot decide to marry a female in order to get his financial needs met. A woman could potentially do this two hundred years ago or two hundred minutes ago.

When I think on the damage that women are allowing their own sons to go through it is enough to make you weep, and I don't say this lightly. Do you realize that for every two children born one of them is a boy and the other a girl? Half the homes on the planet have as its occupant a boy and yet there is no outcry for his pain. There is no outcry by the mother who listens to the voices of media who castigate her little toddler for the same behavior they reward girls. There are no parades by those mothers or women in general to the broader disaster we are driving young male babies towards. No, what we are expected to do is just sit back and ride it out until we see how the dust settles on the gender debate.

For all of you reading this book let me show you what kind of future we are going to golden-parachute into on the debate of equality between the genders. I submit for you as already documented proof, "The Doll Experiment." If you are unfamiliar with The Doll Experiments then know it was used to help settle the landmark case, Brown vs the Board of Education. In this case, the Supreme Court of the United States allowed testimony from Doctor's Kenneth and Mamie Clark who had pioneered an experiment to prove that black children were harmed by racial segregation in the same Public-School system I reference today.

I give you verbatim a summary of the details written by Erin Blakemore of, The History Channel. What I would like you to do as you read over her article is in the place of the black or white dolls substitute male and female dolls. The male doll will be used in place of the black doll and the girl doll in the place of the white doll. It is not the color of the white doll that is important as much as the perceived advantage in an equal system. Today I believe it is time for a new doll experiment. If we ran this experiment across a great many U.S. schools, we would find that boys considered themselves stupid and girls consider them this way also.

We would find that girls consider themselves superior in every nature to males as they have been preached this over the last forty-five years.

The only thing both sides found out is that a belief is stronger than fact or anything else for that matter. You cannot move a people forward or backward without a belief. This same false belief was used to keep the black population as infantile and stupid as possible. But yet in still today, we see these negative subversions for what they are as people cast their vote for the first Black President of the country. Then why are we starting a new round of beliefs fueled by negative Feminist that all boys are stupid and all girls are smart?

The Doll Experiment

How Dolls Helped Win Brown v. Board of Education
Deceptively simple doll tests helped convince the Supreme Court to strike down school segregation.

Dolls are for kids. So why were they in front of the most esteemed judges in the United States?

As they deliberated on Brown v. Board of Education, the landmark 1954 case that eventually overturned "separate-but-equal" segregation in the United States, the Supreme Court Justices contemplated oral arguments and pored over case transcripts. But they also considered black and white baby dolls—unexpected weapons in the plaintiffs' fight against racial discrimination.

The dolls were part of a group of groundbreaking psychological experiments performed by Mamie and Kenneth Clark, a husband-and-wife team of African-American psychologists who devoted their life's work to understanding and helping heal children's racial biases. During the "doll tests," as they're now known, a majority of African-American children showed a preference for dolls with white skin instead of black ones—a consequence, the Clarks argued, of the pernicious effects of segregation.

The Clarks' work, and their testimony in the underlying cases that became Brown v. Board of Education, helped the Supreme Court justices and the nation understand some of the lingering effects of segregation on the very children it affected most.

For the Clarks, the results showed the devastating effects of life in a society that was intolerant of African-Americans. Their experiment, which involved white- and brown-skinned dolls, was deceptively simple. (In a reflection of the racial biases of the time, the Clarks had to paint a white baby doll brown for the tests, since African-American dolls were not yet manufactured.) The children were asked to identify the diapered dolls in a number of ways: the one they wanted to play with, the one that looked "white," "colored," or "Negro," the one that was "good" or "bad." Finally, they were asked to identify the doll that looked most like them.

All of the children tested were black, and all but one group attended segregated schools. Most of the children preferred the white doll to the African-American one. Some of the children would cry and run out of the room when asked to identify which doll looked like them. These results upset the Clarks so much that they delayed publishing their conclusions.

Mamie Clark had connections to the growing legal struggle to overturn segregation—she had worked in the office of one of the lawyers who helped lay the foundation for Brown v. Board of Education. When the NAACP learned of the Clarks' work, they asked them to participate in a case that would later be rolled into the class-action case that went to the Supreme Court. So, Kenneth Clark headed to Clarendon County, South Carolina, to replicate his test with black children there. It was a terrifying experience, he recalled later, especially when his NAACP host was threatened in his presence.

"But we had to test those children," here called. "These children saw themselves as inferior and they accepted the inferiority as part of reality." Thurgood Marshall was eager to use the Clarks' work in the bigger class-action case that would become Brown v. Board of Education, but not everyone was convinced. Attorney Spotswood Robinson told an observer that it was "crazy and insulting to persuade a court of law with examples of crying children and dolls," writes historian Martha Minow. Dr. Kenneth Clark, a New York psychologist and educator, at the North Side Center for Child Development he and his wife founded in Harlem. (Credit: AP Photo)

But the court didn't think so. Kenneth Clark testified at three of the trials and helped write a summary of all five trials' social science testimony that was used in the Supreme Court case. He told judges and juries that African-American children's preference for white dolls represented psychological damage that was reinforced by segregation.

"My opinion is that a fundamental effect of segregation is basic confusion in the individuals and their concepts about themselves conflicting in their self-images," he told the jury in the Briggs case. The sense of inferiority caused by segregation had real, lifelong consequences, he argued—consequences that started before children could even articulate any information about race.

The Clarks' work and testimony were part of a much broader case that combined five cases and covered nearly every aspect of school segregation—and some historians argue that the doll tests played a relatively insignificant part in the court's decision. But echoes of the Clarks' results ring through the unanimous opinion of the Supreme Court justices. Nettie Hunt explaining the meaningful ruling of the Brown v. Board of Education case to her daughter Nickie on the steps of the U.S. Supreme Court. (Credit: Bettmann Archive/Getty Images)

"To separate [black children] from others of similar age and qualifications solely because of their race generates a feeling of inferiority as to their status in the community that may affect their hearts and minds in a way unlikely ever to be undone," wrote Chief Justice Earl Warren in the opinion. The Clarks' work had helped strike down segregation in the United States.

Today, one of the black dolls is on display at the Brown v. Board of Education National Historic Site in Kansas, and integration is the law of the land.

Questions the children were asked in, the Doll Test.

"Show me the doll that you like best or that you'd like to play with,"
"Show me the doll that is the 'nice' doll,"
"Show me the doll that looks 'bad',"

"Give me the doll that looks like a white child,"
"Give me the doll that looks like a colored child,"
"Give me the doll that looks like a Negro child,"
"Give me the doll that looks like you."

-End of Report-

In this most cherished country of personal freedoms leased us by a government on cycles of who is in charge and who may not be; cracks are beginning to form in the lives of demoralized boys. We are beginning to see the steady unraveling's of the purposeful harm done to the human male psyche. I am a combat veteran and I submit to you that there had never been a broader war in all of history before Radicalized Feminist turned female against male.

I am asked frequently why it is that men and women are at each other more negatively than positively in all coupling backgrounds. To those people I say, that's an easy answer. You see to me there has never been a war in all of human history up until the two opposite genders began to oppose one another. Some very crafty snake-like people must have realized that there were only two genders on the planet that were not at war with one another.

This means that all past conflicts were fought as I said before, mainly male against male. But what would happen if you turned the opposite sexes against one another? There could not ever truly be a war unless you turned the opposite gender descendants of the original creation against one another. Now we truly have a global conflict that goes far beyond the battlefield and onto the home field in most countries. You have wives and husbands fighting it out verbally, in front of the children who are forced to decide on which side of the enemy camp they should decide to side with.

In these homes, little girls and boys will be groomed to hate a gender that they are not even the legal age to marry.

By the time they do marry these doctrines will leech out of them like some poorly crafted sieve enough to damage all their hopes and dreams for true love. The un-orderly thought processes that went into a government mandated equality act never anticipated such devastation of a single gender to uplift another. In this countries piecemealed approach at fixing a problem it generated fostered help equivalent to placing bandages on bullet wounds. In evidence, I liken the handling of the government's perceived re-distribution of wealth to its takeover of Iraq and its subsequent turn over to the Iraqi government. This is in sharp contrast to its takeover of Germany during World War II, and its eventual handover of power to the intact German Government.

A lesson that history has repeatedly taught the victor of any domination is that if he retires his support to manage that event then it will cease to exist. Time and time again we have been witnessing to our government imposing then abandoning a twisted system of rule. I fear the government is preparing to abandon women to the same fate they did the Native American, the Black Race and recently the Iraqi citizen.

Between the formalization of the modern Feminist movement and today, women have had a great amount of time to make a coalition course with men over choosing a collision course with them. It would have been far better for men and women both to work out their differences as opposed to a winner-take-all system of equalization. But I would guarantee you that once the global fall of the power of woman hits there will be no monies or support to put the pieces back again.

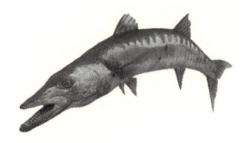

Barracuda Feminist
(The Baby Killer)

"The Barracuda Feminist is on an ethnic cleansing spree. First, she seeks to eradicate man as her perceived enemy, then turn her attention towards his unborn child in an attempt to destroy his lineage."

Charles Rivers

I could place just one word for this entire chapter and call it a day; heartless. But the pro-abortion feminist is much more than cold-blooded. For the abortion feminist who pushes baby killings as a means of liberty for women knows nothing of freedom. The last time a woman was sold such a raw bill of goods like abortion she lost her house and home over a shiny apple on a forbidden tree from and a snake in the grass. This avenue of thinking is little more than another double standard of stupidity set to music. The modern identity of abortion to allow a woman not to miss a day at work does stem from a humanitarian point of view but from a war-crimes dogmatic stance. The medical wing of the then 1940's president of Germany took direct orders from Hitler to carry out abortions and mercy killings.

Those of you who are familiar with history know that Adolph Hitler was not only a self-proclaimed war general but the President of Germany. Mr. Hitler was hardly a humanitarian and as a Nazi, certainly not a feminist.

The Nazis were not "pro-choice", but they were not "anti-abortion" either. The Nazis believed that a woman's body belonged to the State, and the State would decide what to do with it. The Nazis did not allow abortion for healthy "Aryan" German women, but demanded and forced abortion upon women deemed "un-Aryan" (i.e. Jews, Gypsies, Slavs, etc.) and "Aryan" German women who were thought to be feeble-minded, or have hereditary diseases.

Note- *In the United States, black children are aborted at more than three times the rate of white children; Hispanic children are aborted at one and a half times the rate. Whatever the intentions of Planned Parenthood, abortion is eliminating an incommensurate number of minority children.* Statistics @ *Abort73.com*

The ideology of the Nazis was based on social Darwinism that held unreservedly to the notion of the survival of the fittest, at both the level of the individual as well as the level of entire peoples and states. This notion claimed to have natural law on its side. All opposing religious and humanitarian views would ultimately prove to be unnatural. A people could only prove its worth in the long run in this ongoing "struggle for survival", if they promoted the best and, if necessary, eliminated those that weakened them.

Moreover, only people as racially pure as possible could maintain the "struggle for existence". To maintain or improve the Nordic-Germanic race, therefore, the laws of eugenics or the (bio logistically oriented) "racial hygiene" would have to be strictly observed, that is, the promotion of the "genetically healthy" and the elimination of the "sick". All those with hereditary illnesses or who were severely mentally and physically handicapped were classified as "lives unworthy of life" (lebensunwertes Leben).

They would, in terms of natural selection, be "eliminated". This form of eugenics was eventually the basis of the National Socialist genetic health policy which was elevated to the rank of state doctrine.

In 1929 Hitler said at the Nazi Party Conference in Nuremberg, "that an average annual removal of 700,000-800,000 of the weakest of a million babies meant an increase in the power of the nation and not a weakening". In doing so, he was able to draw upon a scientific argument that transferred the Darwinian theory of natural selection to human beings and, through the concept of racial hygiene, formulated the "Utopia" of "human selection" as propounded by Alfred Ploetz, the founder of German racial hygiene.

As early as 1895, he demanded that human offspring should not: be left to the chance encounter of a drunken moment. [...] If nevertheless, it turns out that the newborn baby is a weak and misbegotten child, the medical council, which decides on citizenship for the community, should prepare a gentle death for it, say, using a little dose of morphine.

In 1935 Hitler also announced at the Nuremberg Nazi Party to the Reich Medical Leader Gerhard Wagner that he should aim to "eliminate the incurably insane", at the latest, in the event of a future war." The elimination of "undesirable elements" was implemented under the term "euthanasia" at the beginning of the Second World War. Petitions from parents of disabled children to Hitler's Chancellery (KDF) that asked for their children to be given "mercy killing" were used as a justifiable excuse and to demonstrate external demand.

Aktion T4 (German, pronounced [akˈtsioːn teː fiːɐ]) was a postwar name for mass murder through involuntary euthanasia in Nazi Germany.[4][b] The name T4 is an abbreviation of Tiergartenstraße 4, a street address of the Chancellery department set up in the spring of 1940, in the Berlin borough of Tiergarten, which recruited and paid personnel associated with T4. Certain German physicians were authorized to select patients "deemed incurably sick, after most critical medical examination" and then administer to them a "mercy death" (Gnadentod).

In October 1939, Adolf Hitler signed a "euthanasia note", backdated to 1 September 1939, which authorized his physician Karl Brandt and Reichsleiter Philipp Bouhler to implement the program.

The killings took place from September 1939 until the end of the war in 1945; from 275,000 to 300,000 people were killed in psychiatric hospitals in Germany and Austria, occupied Poland and the Protectorate of Bohemia and Moravia (now the Czech Republic). The number of victims was originally recorded as 70,273 but this number has been increased by the discovery of victims listed in the archives of the former East Germany.

About half of those killed were taken from church-run asylums, often with the approval of the Protestant or Catholic authorities of the institutions. The Holy See announced on 2 December 1940 that the policy was contrary to the natural and positive Divine law and that "the direct killing of an innocent person because of mental or physical defects is not allowed" but the declaration was not upheld by some Catholic authorities in Germany.

In the summer of 1941, protests were led in Germany by the Bishop of Münster, Clemens von Galen, whose intervention led to "the strongest, most explicit and most widespread protest movement against any policy since the beginning of the Third Reich", according to Richard J. Evans. Several reasons have been suggested for the killings, including eugenics, compassion, reducing suffering, racial hygiene and saving money.

Physicians in German and Austrian asylums continued many of the practices of Aktion T4 until the defeat of Germany in 1945, in spite of its official cessation in August 1941. The informal continuation of the policy led to 93,521 "beds emptied" by the end of 1941.

Technology developed under Aktion T4 was taken over by the medical division of the Reich Interior Ministry, particularly the use of lethal gas to kill large numbers of people, along with the personnel of Aktion T4, who participated in Operation Reinhard.[23] The program was authorized by Hitler but the killings have since come to be viewed as murders in Germany. The number of people killed was about 200,000 in Germany and Austria, with about 100,000 victims in other European countries.

In knowing this information I always encourage women to watch where they are taking their cues to abort from. So far I can name no sense of decency from a gender who claims to be more decent and loving than the men they despise and try to undermine. In fact, the more women invent ways to hurt males society begins to view masculinity as a victim of Oppressive Fanatical Feminism.

This and this alone is why women will not win in the next general election. The more American and world society begins to wake up to the dusted off philosophies of a dictators, separatist or racist sexism in women they will flee their support to this demonic cause. Until women fight for the rights of both over the rights of self she will continue to lose allies. Until there is a real and not pretended sense of equality she will find herself on the outs.

What's good for the goose is good for the gander. What is good for a man is equally good for a woman; or, what a man can have or do, so can a woman have or do. This comes from an earlier proverb, "What's sauce for the goose is sauce for the gander."

-Dictionary.com-

Spreading the Sauce

If a woman has a right to abort a child than so does her mate to which the child's DNA originated from. That's right, it takes two parents to make that child, not one. So if rights are equal then the father should have the same right in the say so of abortion or life. But no one would ever want to hear of such a thing. They would say that this is the body of a woman and her decision to choose. Actually, this too is a fallacy of great proportion. Sex is the only exercise where two people go into a room and come out with three people.

We can debate the semantics all year long as to whether it is a child after the heartbeat or before it. But when the woman has shared her body with another man it is no longer just her body but three peoples bodies. Yes, she has authority over her body but she willingly shared it with the man. Then she willingly shared her body with his unborn child. But if she follows the natural double-standard of feminism she will renege on the shared body concept and call it her body only along with a single-minded position to abort. There is no industry in the world in which someone would willingly hire you, allow you in a group or an intimate setting and allow you to back out in such a way.

The difference with feminism is that it sets too wide a chasm between love and sex. It encourages women to explore sex the way a man would but without planning the consequences. Never before in the history of civilization or tomorrow will a man get pregnant. So to suggest that both are equal in a sexual sense is foolhardy.

The only time men and women are totally equal is when a woman is not pregnant. Every little boy and every little girl share in common being without a child. It is when a woman exercises her free will to mate does she change this equation. In all but a few cases of pregnancy, it was by choice. Before that moment both sexes were born without being pregnant. Let us speak about times where a woman feels that a man's body is not truly his but hers.

Another's Body as Ownership

"It is not the males of today that need to be taught about the gift of equality, but the females."

Charles Rivers

In any relationship, a woman shares with a man she considers his body hers to do with as she pleases and not his alone. Just as soon as a woman gets into a relationship with a man she begins to change the wardrobe on his body. The second thing she does is change his hairstyle to suit her preference. She changes out his body wash and cologne so she as well as her friends find the approval of his scent. She changes out his shoes and his personality to suit her needs. Now all these things together are small forms of using someone else's body as if it were yours but they don't compare to the next examples.

A woman in a relationship with a man will control his sexual desires. She will remove any pornographic magazines or movies from his house that was there before she arrived. Is that bad, not yet, but I'm getting there.

She then lowers the incidents where she has sex with him as compared to her romantic phase of the relationship. In effect, most women are taught to do the old bait-and-switch when it comes to men. Whatever gets you in the door and a ring for security reasons is worth pretending you enjoy for the short-run. After she reduces having sex with him she begins to use sex as a weapon or reward, the carrot or stick motivation method. Finally, she reduces sex from a few times a month to twice a year or not at all. Wait for it, wait for it. As a result of a fertile man being stuck in a no sex relationship he seeks gratification outside of the home.

Yes, women lose their homes by their own understandings of what a man is and what he is not. With the separation of affection, he begins to pursue people who are not of reputable means away from the home. Within the bodies of these persons awaits diseases such as herpes, Aids and syphilis. When she does decide to have sex with him again these diseases will be transmitted back to her.

At that time you will not hear the argument that his body is his. No, what you will here is that your body is not yours alone, we are in a relationship together and what you do can affect both of us. She will tell him that you could have killed me doing something so stupid. In a relationship, there is no such thing as your body is yours solely. If you wanted your body to your self then you should have stayed to yourself.

In a relationship, if a husband drinks and drives with his wife and baby in the car he can't stand on the argument that his body is his own and risk it with her in the car. Nope, everybody in that car is going to be missing a body at this rate. So the next time you hear the argument that it is her body then unless you got pregnant the same way that Jesus mother did it is with the help of a man. Till this day I could never understand why a group of people who referred to themselves as militant feminist gets dressed in the most attractive clothing and pretend to be Miss. Susie Homemaker on Friday night just to get laid by those little men they say they hate the most.

Mean what You Say

I like to speak a moment on the bedrock of radical feminist theology; which is, use a forked tongue when you speak. If you are talking to a feminist in any situation there will be no facts to stick to as she will weave her way in and out of the situations you try to pin her down to. A radical feminist beats the drum that all females are smarter than men. I like to explore this strength of the moment right here and now. If a woman is intrinsically smarter than men, then how did the woman who wishes to get an abortion get pregnant in the first place? The feminist will bemoan. "it is because he tricked the woman into getting pregnant." We are back in a circular logic pattern with this question. How can a man who is presumed to be dumb trick a much intelligent woman into such a thing?

Well, it was an accident and that is why she got pregnant. This too is one of the largest cover-your-backside lies to come out of feminism. First thing, women enjoy sex just as much as men do although many are afraid to admit it unless they are in an online chatroom where they can remain anonymous. Secondly, there is a drive to sexual arousal in most young people that is fueled by the fantasy of risk sex. Women just like men find heightened excitement with the risk of getting pregnant through intercourse or without using a condom. To further dismiss the case of superiority between the genders I have included a list of how many stages you would have to miss to even consider getting an abortion as a feminist woman.

18 Alphabets to Preventing Unwanted Pregnancies other than Abortion

a. **Abstinence**- The average liberated woman who claims to hate all men must find it funny when she wakes up beside a total stranger after sex. If her behavior follows the logic of a separatist and a racist throughout this book I would have to say she is in keeping with the slavemaster who would hate slaves but sleep with female slaves over his own wife. Women who have sex with men and claim to hate all men are as confusing as the sun rising in the East and set in the North to me. The reason a lot of people chose not to use any of these methods is that it will either hurt their body as they will the struggling unborn fetus at the abortionist clinic or they feel they are too cumbersome. Others feel that they either take too much time or allow the arousal of someone you need only for sex to diminish.

b. **Birth Control Implant**
99% Effective
Can cost $0 to $1,300
Lasts Up To 5 years

c. **IUD**
99% Effective
Can cost $0 to $1,300
Lasts Up To 3-12 years

d. **Birth Control Shot**
94% Effective
Can cost $0 to $100
Get every 3 months

e. **Birth Control Vaginal Ring**
91% Effective
Can cost $0 to $200
Replace monthly

f. **Birth Control Patch**
    91% Effective
    Can cost $0 to $150
    Replace weekly

g. **Birth Control Pill**
    91% Effective
    Can cost $0 to $50
    Take daily

h. **Condom**
    85% Effective
    Can cost $0 to $2
    Use every time

I. **Internal Condom**
    79% Effective
    Can cost $0 to $3
    Use every time

J. **Diaphragm**
    88% Effective
    Can cost $0 to $75
    Use every time

k. **Birth Control Sponge**
    76-88% Effective
    Can cost $0 to $15

l. **Cervical Cap**
    71-86% Effective
    Can cost $0 to $90
    Use every time

m. **Spermicide**
    71% Effective

Can cost $0 to $8
Use every time

n. **Fertility Awareness (FAMs)**
76-88% Effective
Can cost $0 to $20
Use daily

o. **Withdrawal (Pull Out Method)**
78% Effective
Cost $0
Use Every Time

p. **Breastfeeding as Birth Control**
98% Effective
Cost $0
Do every 4-5 hours

q. **Sterilization (Tubal Ligation)**
99% Effective
Can cost $0 to $6,000
Lasts for Life

r. **Vasectomy**
99% Effective
Can cost $0 to $1,000
Lasts for life

As I said at the beginning of these statistics as a feminist you can always leave men alone. You will find that they have other means as well to enjoy the abilities of sex. Plus you can always use the trusty vibrator that you hide in the corner top of your dresser. With regular cleaning, you can avoid giving even your own self a yeast infection.

According to WHO, (World Health Organization) every year in the world there are an estimated 40-50 million abortions? This corresponds to approximately 125,000 abortions per day.

In 2015, 638,169 legal induced abortions were reported to CDC from 49 reporting areas. The abortion rate for 2015 was 11.8 abortions per 1,000 women aged 15–44 years, and the abortion ratio was 188 abortions per 1,000 live births.

Smith said that since 1973, when the Supreme Court handed down its decision in Roe v. Wade, there have been "well over" 54 million abortions. The Guttmacher Institute has tracked roughly 49.3 million abortions through 2008.Mar 18, 2012

According to WHO statistics, the risk rate for unsafe abortion is 1/270; according to other sources, unsafe abortion is responsible for at least 8% of maternal deaths. Worldwide, 48% of all induced abortions are unsafe. The British Medical Bulletin reported in 2003 that 70,000 women a year die from unsafe abortion.

Before the U.S. Supreme Court decision Roe v. Wade decriminalized abortion nationwide in 1973, abortion was already legal in several states, but the decision imposed a uniform framework for state legislation on the subject.

Girls under the age of 18 must get written permission from a parent or guardian before being allowed an abortion.

• Total number of abortions in the U.S. 1973-2013: 56.5 million+
• 219 abortions per 1,000 live births (according to the Centers for Disease Control)
• Abortions per year: 1.058 million
• Abortions per day: 2,899
• Abortions per hour: 120
• 1 abortion every 30 seconds

Roughly fifty million deaths have been perpetrated in all of the wars in history, but abortion makes women higher killers.

1.72 billion Abortions worldwide in the last 40 years

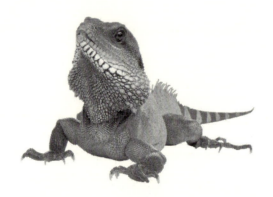

Iguana Feminist
(The Female Pedophile)

"After the dust has settled, society is going to realize that there are more Iguana Feminist hiding in the shadows then there are victims to have come forward."

Charles Rivers

In this chapter, we are going to be bringing truth to darkness concerning women's overt and covert sexuality practices. I want to reveal that in the area of sexuality that females are truly just as nasty as they claim males to be. When it comes to pornography, sexual harassment, child molestation or adultery women are truly making strides. The first truth that society does not hold to be self-evident is that women enjoy pornography. When I say pornography, I don't mean those nasty little dime novels with the bare-chested lumber-jack on the cover. Sure, these books may appear innocuous on the surface but some are trashier than the worst xxx porn movies and available at the dresser of every mom when her daughter is home alone.

Sure, the billion-dollar romance novel industry sees a larger portion of college-age black women as their readers but that same demographic is not recognized in its award-winning writer, go figure. The first thing we will try to force into the open is the modern-day feminist closeted pornographic habits. The following information is given after an extensive click by click viewership of women's online porn habits. The numbers are in on the Iguana Feminist and it would seem that she is not as wholesome as she publicly appears. It seems that her most clicked upon videos in any given search are for lesbianism.

That's right, even more than men; women prefer two women having sex, or lesbian sex as a turn-on. This number really peaks if you relate it to women over the age of forty-five years of age. Also, the numbers show that women actually view these videos longer than men when online. The second category that women shockingly prefer is rough sex. Duh…what?

For as long as we can remember and until today all you hear on television is that pornography paints women in a negative light and that pornography cause's harm to women. We were told that it promotes violence against women. We were told that most women prefer romantic sex where there is an equality of love. Lie! Women prefer rough sex in a closeted way but profess something different in public not to appear as perverted as the men they demonize.

These collected data numbers show that women use their cell phones more for watching porn then men do. I guess it's easier to hit the delete button on a smartphone than it is on a desktop computer. The biggest shock from the decency police at Feminism Headquarters is that one of the highest viewed categories was male on male gay porn. Oh no, say it isn't so. Yes, women get aroused watching two men go at it as reported by Pornhub and X-Hamster statistics.

Other high porn films viewed by women were threesomes, gangbangs, teen 18+ double penetrations, and bondage along with ebony sex. I will do you the favor at leaving it right there before you need a vomit bag for the other categories of female porn fantasies that are hidden. So now that we see there is an equality of filth let's move to the child molestation.

I have attached but one story of many that entail modern day Feminist in a country where sex is easily available to the Radical Liberated Feminist choosing to have it with children instead. I would ask that the general reading public forget the agreement concerning women and bipolar disorder as men are not granted the same excuses in the case of pedophilia. Nor are they imprisoned the same way, for the same exact crime.

North Carolina woman who worked at church day school arrested in child pornography case; victims ages 2-3

APRIL 5, 2019, BY CNN WIRE

Greensboro (WGHP) — A woman was charged Friday with indecent liberties in a child pornography investigation while she was working at a Greensboro church's day school, Homeland Security Investigations reports.

Alyson Brooke Saunders, 23, who worked at Fellowship Presbyterian Church's Fellowship Day School in Greensboro, was arrested Friday morning and charged with six counts of first-degree sexual exploitation of a minor, two counts of sex offense on a child by an adult, four counts of indecent liberties with a child and two counts of crimes against nature. She is being held under a $1 million bond.

The photos and videos depict indecent liberties against child victims that are between the ages of 2 to 3, according to warrants. The abuse allegedly happened at the daycare, some of it on a changing room table. The crimes against nature charge involved a dog. The remaining details listed on the warrants are too graphic to report. Saunders allegedly forwarded the images to someone in Great Britain. Fellowship Day School operates both pre-school and after-school programs. Saunders was terminated from the school after her arrest Friday.

Saunders' name was brought into the case when Homeland Security Investigations in London arrested a person on child pornography charges overseas and learned the suspect had communicated with Saunders over the Internet. HSI London then contacted HSI Winston-Salem in February. Special agents reached out to Saunders, who agreed to a consensual interview and allowed agents to preview her electronic media. In March, she admitted to exploiting and producing pornography of minor children, Homeland Security reports. Forensic analysis confirmed that she produced and disseminated child pornography, according to HSI.

-End of Report-

Most young boys that have been prematurely touched sexually suffer in silence right through their teen years and adulthood. Because these boys have been either penetrated or forced to penetrate by his perpetrator, he ultimately considers himself to be a weaker man in the society of men. In his imagination, only a lesser male would allow such a vulnerable thing to happen.

This one insult against a boy's pride is hard to explain to a mother who was in herself designed to be penetrated. Even in the opposite case of a woman exposing herself to her victim, he takes on the mantle of an effeminate shame. He reasons, why would that woman pursue me over other males if she did not feel me to be a weaker person who would not tell? What did she see in my personality that I did not and that others will surely attack?

I have dealt with an innumerous number of men who tell me their horror stories of sexual abuse and mental shame. Molestation of boys today is not merely a male on male crime. If you believe this to be a penetration crime then don't fool yourself. This is a crime of theft that is perpetuated from generation to generation. If molestation goes on in a home, you can bet that it is capable of traveling to the molested boys future home through him. It may not show up in the case of him reenacting this heinous crime but his personality towards his own children and lover will not be anything to write home about.

So, what are we looking for when it comes to female perpetrators of this crime? Do we turn to the evening news to watch yet another female school teacher being paraded for engaging in sex with her minor student? No, the problem is much more expansive than that. There are sisters, nieces, aunts, mothers, grandmothers, and especially female friends who molest boys in secret.

There are boys who have been molested in silence who keep that tragedy under wraps until their dying day. If that were not bad enough there are places outside of the home that the molested boy is virtually raped by his own babysitter. Just as girls who face being touched against their will, there can be a sense of shame, guilt, and remorse by boys as well. Shame for the immature sexual mind does not merely come from being touched too early in your life-cycle. There are a myriad number of different issues that are affected after this event has long since passed. What most of these cases of molestation involve is vulnerability. Secondly, they involve the trust I laid out for you earlier in this book.

That trust is the societal belief that woman is nicer and not as sexual as men. This learned trust is a false belief that women do not prefer sex as much as men. That trust on its face is about as real as Santa Claus riding a unicorn on a gumdrop trail. Don't let them fool you; women are nasty all day long. I guarantee as you go about your daily life that you do not pass people having sex on the public sidewalks of your neighborhood street. Nope, most adults intentionally have sex indoors and out of sight of the general public. Why, because we have been taught that it is a shameful act if viewed in public. We are taught that this is a completely private act.

This training is what the female molester teaches her victim. She seeks to impart to him that what happens behind closed doors, stays behind closed doors. In order to avoid detection, punishment, and retribution, she must gain trust, privacy and anonymity. She must gain your son's trust over time in order to have him all to herself under that same hidden sexless guise.

Another thing that is important to the she-molester is to gain the vulnerable boy's participation.

If you are not going to be a willing participant in this insanity then peer pressure or the threat of retribution will be exerted upon you. Whether the molested boy is an active participant or not usually will not prevent this horrible crime from taking place. In some of these thefts of innocence cases children that have been prepared by a parent come out much better than the unprepared.

They readied kids are immediately motivated to, get up, run like hell and tell. But this is not true for all cases of child molestation. Most of these children are chosen for these stealthy rendezvous specifically because they are perceived not to fight but to freeze up in the face of adversity. You will notice in this chapter a return to the Greek love levels I explained to you in the first portion of this book. The only difference now is that this list is reversed as it pertains to a child's growth cycle.

During a human boy's growth cycle, his psyche is graduated into three separate and distinct love categories in order to give him a healthy body image and upbringing. In the first psychological building stage, he is born to the **Agape Love** state of mind. In this stage of a child's growth and development, we are equivalent to what our grandmothers call, her little angel. We don't have the rational discernment to know whether something is right or wrong as long as it is presented by someone in authority over us. We don't carry animosity or animus for any particular person, race, gender or nationality. These and many other hates, haunts, and failings will be taught in our next level of growth.

The second stage of growth is what all infants fall into at or around the age of six years of age being a **Philia Love** state of mind. In this love stage, we learn to widen our circle of trust beyond our home to other neighborhoods and certainly other school students. This is the mental stage of learning and discerning of what a friend is and what he or she is not. This is the stage of psychological growth that the molester intends to target if they have not already in the Agape stage of growth. As Philia toddlers we go about meeting people to make as many unnecessary friends without the filter of experience will allow us.

Our final stage of growth comes around the age of puberty and is best referred to as our **Erotic Love** blossoming. Most young people have arrived at this stage of puberty become naturally sexualized in order to continue on the human species. The danger is what happens before they are at the mental stage of wrapping up what sex really means as well as what it really means to them. When an infant, toddler or young person is touched in a molestation fashion a jump to the Erotic stage of love arrives long before it can be appreciated for what it really is.

Something intimate that would have been mutually accepted at a later time in life becomes something dirty. The molested boy may feel sexualized feelings that they never knew they had before. They may feel that they are gay even though they were manipulated by the opposite gender. They will wonder why they were targeted by this adult woman; believing falsely that they put out a particular sexualized vibe.

They will receive the false understanding that sex is something that is dirty and is only used to please the molester over the molested. Like touching a hot stove, the mind of the molested they can never go back to the moment before this cruelty occurred. Like a victim of rape, they will most assuredly feel unclean and damaged mentally by the event. In the rarest of cases, they will tell a parent or someone closest to them. But with the inner guilt and remorse, they feel which is strengthened by the molester his secret remains. I attach this story from the Scientific American on the statistics of boys being molested by both genders.

Sexual Victimization by Women Is More Common Than Previously Known

A new study gives a portrait of female perpetrators

By Lara Stemple, Ilan H. Meyer on October 10, 2017

Take a moment and picture an image of a rapist. Without a doubt, you are thinking about a man. Given our pervasive cultural understanding that perpetrators of sexual violence are nearly always men, this makes sense. But this assumption belies the reality, revealed in our study of large-scale federal agency surveys, that women are also often perpetrators of sexual victimization.

In 2014, we published a study on the sexual victimization of men, finding that men were much more likely to be victims of sexual abuse than was thought. To understand who was committing the abuse, we next analyzed four surveys conducted by the Bureau of Justice Statistics (BJS) and the Centers for Disease Control and Prevention (CDC) to glean an overall picture of how frequently women were committing sexual victimization.

The results were surprising. For example, the CDC's nationally representative data revealed that over one year, men and women were equally likely to experience nonconsensual sex, and most male victims reported female perpetrators. Over their lifetime, 79 percent of men who were "made to penetrate" someone else (a form of rape, in the view of most researchers) reported female perpetrators. Likewise, most men who experienced sexual coercion and unwanted sexual contact had female perpetrators.

We also pooled four years of the National Crime Victimization Survey (NCVS) data and found that 35 percent of male victims who experienced rape or sexual assault reported at least one female perpetrator. Among those who were raped or sexually assaulted by a woman, 58 percent of male victims and 41 percent of female victims reported that the incident involved a violent attack, meaning the female perpetrator hit, knocked down or otherwise attacked the victim, many of whom reported injuries.

And, because we had previously shown that nearly one million incidents of sexual victimization happen in our nation's prisons and jails each year, we knew that no analysis of sexual victimization in the U.S. would be complete without a look at sexual abuse happening behind bars. We found that, contrary to assumptions, the biggest threat to women serving time does not come from male corrections staff. Instead, female victims are more than three times more likely to experience sexual abuse by other women inmates than by male staff.

Also, surprisingly, women inmates are more likely to be abused by other inmates than are male inmates, disrupting the long-held view that sexual violence in prison is mainly about men assaulting men. In juvenile corrections facilities, female staff is also a much more significant threat than male staff; more than nine in ten juveniles who reported staff sexual victimization were abused by a woman.

Our findings might be critically viewed as an effort to upend a women's rights agenda that focuses on the sexual threat posed by men. To the contrary, we argue that male-perpetrated sexual victimization remains a chronic problem, from the schoolyard to the White House. In fact, 96 percent of women who report rape or sexual assault in the NCVS were abused by men. In presenting our findings, we argue that a comprehensive look at sexual victimization, which includes male perpetration and adds female perpetration, is consistent with feminist principles in important ways.

For example, the common one-dimensional portrayal of women as harmless neutered caregivers reinforces outdated gender stereotypes. This keeps us from seeing women as complex human beings, able to wield power, even in misguided or violent ways. And, the assumption that men are always perpetrators and never victims reinforce unhealthy ideas about men and their supposed invincibility. These hyper-masculine ideals can reinforce aggressive male attitudes and, at the same time, callously stereotype male victims of sexual abuse as "failed men."

Other gender stereotypes prevent effective responses, such as the trope that men are sexually insatiable. Aware of the popular misconception that, for men, all sex is welcome, male victims often feel too embarrassed to report sexual victimization. If they do report it, they are frequently met with a response that assumes no real harm was done.

Women abused by other women are also an overlooked group; these victims discover that most services are designed for women victimized by men. Behind bars, we found that sexual minorities were 2-3 times more likely to be sexually victimized by staff members than straight inmates. This is particularly alarming as our related research found that sexual minorities, especially lesbian and bisexual women, are much more likely to be incarcerated to begin with.

In addition to the risk faced by sexual minorities, the U.S. disproportionately incarcerates people who are black, Latino/a, low-income, or mentally ill, putting these populations at risk of abuse. Detained juveniles experience particularly high rates of sexual victimization, and young people outside of the system are also at risk. A recent study of youth found, strikingly, that females comprise 48 percent of those who self-reported committing rape or attempted rape at age 18-19.

Professionals in mental health, social work, public health, and criminal justice often downplay female perpetration. But in fact, victims of female-perpetrated sexual violence suffer emotional and psychological harm, just like victims of male-perpetrated abuse. And when professionals fail to take victimization by women seriously, this only compound victims' suffering by minimizing the harm they experience.

Researchers also find that female perpetrators have often been previously sexually victimized themselves. Women who commit sexual victimization are more likely to have an extensive history of sexual abuse, with more perpetrators and at earlier ages than those who commit other crimes. Some women commit sexual victimization alongside abusive male co-perpetrators. These patterns of gender-based violence must be understood in order to reach the troubled women who harm others.

To thoroughly dismantle sexual victimization, we must grapple with its many complexities, which require attention to all victims and perpetrators, regardless of their sex. This inclusive framing need not and should not come at the expense of gender-sensitive approaches, which take into account the ways in which gender norms influence women and men in different or disproportionate ways.

Male-perpetrated sexual victimization finally came to public attention after centuries of denial and indifference, thanks to women's rights advocates and the anti-rape movement. Attention to sexual victimization perpetrated by women should be understood as a necessary next step in continuing and expanding upon this important legacy.

-End of Story-

The molestation survivor is usually on a fast track to adulthood following the event. He is now actually an adult trapped in the body of a child. He is at a loss to deal with his own peer group. Being exposed to sex far too early before he was mentally prepared for it drops the child immediately from Agape Love level to the basement of loves or Erotic Love in one-fell-swoop. If you have a child that has been molested by a woman you may begin to notice that he is acting strangely in their dress habits as opposed to the day before.

He may no longer want to be undressed by you or in your presence at this early stage of growth and development. Where you would easily have given him a bath the day before he will most certainly give you the suggestion that he can do it himself. Mother's and Father's both erroneously confuse these requests for space with their child maturing earlier in life. They see this as a source of pride for the child as opposed to a cry of desperation.

In some instances, the boy may refuse to bathe at all in a futile attempt not to touch the same parts that someone did in a bad way. In some cases, the boy may not wipe his own back-side after using the toilet. Children of molestation refuse to change in front of other boys or refuse classes like gym, track, and other physical sports. If your child has been molested by a particular person, they may not tell you up front, but they will say things like, "I don't like going to such and such's house anymore." Now, this is not concrete proof in all cases but keep those feelers out there.

If your child immediately changes his habits prior to the age that this behavior should grow naturally then anticipate something is up. In some cases, the molester of your son may be another girl the age of your son or slightly older. There is no hard and fast rule that the molester of a kid has to be an adult. Since I have been coaching grownups for over two decades now, I have learned to notice the signs of childhood molestation exhibited by grown men. Some show noticeable signs and others have lived such a life of masking it that they take on dual personalities that even conceal the truth from themselves.

Other adult males that have been molested end up becoming homosexual, but not in all cases. There again is no hard and fast rule that if you get molested you may become gay. There are many boys now men that have grown up to start their own families through heterosexual marriages.

The danger to the molested boy is that they feel they are effeminate dominated and in a twisted sense feeling that they may have enjoyed a perverted sense of being touched when they could have run away. Some males who get married later on in life to women carry this burden in secret with them feeling that their wives won't understand. In fact, if you are a man reading this book right now this could have happened to you and it became your little dirty secret in order to maintain your sanity and sense of masculinity.

As a teacher to the molested boy, we want to understand how to deal with his problem. You do not have to be molested to understand his feelings. You have all of the training you will need in life to make your son whole despite what he has gone through. If you doubt this, use your workplace attitude for clues on how to deal with the molested boy.

The focus in healing him is not on someone you know that has been molested but someone who has shared a loss with you. For you see the greatest tragedy of the molested boy, is that he has had something stolen or lost that he can never really recover. You have coworkers that have experienced a death in the family, this too is a loss. You have had coworkers who have gone through a bitter divorce, this is a loss.

> *"Most people fail at what they are good at."*
>
> Charles Rivers

You have had friends whose sons were deployed to combat environments and did not make it back home, this again is a loss. You comforted those people and felt true empathy for them. Now the only thing you have to do is put your feelers out there when something like this tragedy strikes your home. Don't run away from the acknowledgment of it for this won't make it go away. If your fellow coworker just had her house burn down overnight would you pretend it never existed? How many people at your job would gather clothes? How many others would gather monies and replacement items until she got on her feet again?

> *"Usually, whatever service you offer outside of your home is the service that your home will be truly lacking."*
>
> Charles Rivers

In some homes, the mother and father have become aware of this heinous event taking place but do little after the occurrence has been corrected through the arrest of the perpetrator. They walk on egg-shells around their own child and try not to be alone with their boys. They treat him as if every day for the rest of his life he was being molested. In this way, the molestation never has a chance to heal in the minds of the survivor. The molested boy is a different case, a special case and no longer one of the regular kids. In a sense, he is now more mature than the rest of his peers for he has experienced an adult event while they are still playing hopscotch and Barrel of Monkeys.

Like the physically abused child, he will most certainly be hiding behind the mask of perfectionism over apathy. The perfectionistic child no longer wants to be abused so he avoids all instances of correction by living a self-corrective existence. The molested boy may shy back at your tender touches and glances that before were once reassuring. At other times, he may retreat backward into infantile behaviors such as bed-wetting and the like. He may run to your arms and never want to leave your protective site. He will for sure begin to take a noticeable dive in his school grades.

As a parent, you will fall into the false belief as many parent's do that, he is afraid of the school work when he is afraid of a particular person. The dreams themselves of the molested child will be forever changed due to this cruel hoax of twisted love. When I say dreams, I do not mean those that occur at nighttime for those will change shortly to nightmares. The dreams I reference are those of career and long-lasting goals.

If you cannot step up and be the guide for the molested boy his later life will reflect his current tragedy. The molested boy faces a normalized tragic life of drug abuse, alcoholism, sexual abuse or molesting other children as was done to him. These acts of violence are in actuality lower quality drugs that give him the dopamine rush he needs to calm down the memory of loss. It gives him the pleasure that once pored freely from his spirit like a Fountain of Youth.

> *"Through being introduces to pornography or touched in silence where no adult is allowed to follow, the overly-sexualized molested boy cries out for attention with each victim he passes his newfound addiction to"*
>
> Charles Rivers

I have assisted in coaching grown men back to wellness who have lived through this egregiousness nightmare.

I have brought them ever closer to healing by teaching them how to forgive their abuser. Without forgiveness, we become permanently trapped in a vicious cycle of anger, hatred and blame for all parties involved. Here is one example I give you of the long-term damage of innocent molested boys without true healing. One morning a woman who heard me speaking on my radio program called me up for counseling between her husband and I. She spoke briefly in a rushed but painful fashion over the phone for about fifteen minutes. I told her that if she got her husband in the room, I would be willing to work with the two of them.

I did not know whether she would go through with our meet but she raised the bar that day and leapt headlong into recovery. That same afternoon she had him in place and relaxed; she came to life. I mean she opened up and ran her husband down for ten minutes straight without breathing. I am quite sure it seemed an eternity for him but he didn't budge. He acted as if he was no longer phased by her brow-beating. In his eyes, this was her usual manner and nothing to get upset about. She finished her diatribe by saying that if I couldn't fix their situation then she would be willing to get a divorce.

Wow, no pressure there. If I couldn't come through huh? Well, it was her lucky day that I never shrank from any challenge, and especially not this one. Let me give you some background information on that story as she recanted it to me. She said that she was tired of changing her daughter's diapers all the time. She said that her husband never helped her as an equal co-parent. She went on to say that it feels almost as if she was raising two children instead of one.

Once she stopped for a minute to gain her breath and composure, I assured that she had said everything she had wanted to. But I was not convinced that their problems were so cut and dry concerning changing a baby's diaper. So, I informed her that I didn't think that this was their issue. Now, remember, I had only been listening to her for a little over nine minutes of a relationship they had for over nine years and with a recent arrival of a daughter to the family.

Keep in mind that she was willing to walk out on her husband for refusing to change his own girl's diapers. In these situations, I typically find that the innocent party in a relationship is the one who is being demonized and yelled at; although not in all degrees. I stopped her before she started in on him again and said we are going to allow him to speak now.

She looked at me as if I didn't know what the hell I was doing. The look in her eyes said, "What do you mean by letting him speak. He is the guilty party here and you need to tell him how to step up to the plate and become a modern diaper-changing dad." I said I believe we have to let him talk for a while now.

I told her that I know that I have only known you guys for about nine minutes and you have been with each other for nine years but this thing you profess is not the root of your problem. This is not the main issue as far as your daughter or you are concerned. I said let him tell you what he has been trying to say to you over the entire length of your marriage. Do you believe me mam, I inquired of her?

She looked at me again as if I had lost my last mind. How could I be already expecting to pass judgment on their problem without knowing them for several weeks? You don't need weeks in some surface cases where an outside participant can see what any loving person is blinded to. I equate this exercise with, not being able to see the forest for the tree's syndrome. At this point, she was willing to humor me and allow at my behest a move forward. I then turned towards her husband and asked him to tell her.

Tell her I said. Tell her what you have been hiding from her as a secret this entire nine-years. At once, everyone in the room to include the stenographer of the meeting became eerily silent and motionless. Could he be hiding something that she never picked up on in their nine years of intimacy? Was he hiding an affair or worse? He looked at me, with a trapped expression, then looked at her and finally back at me. Again, I exclaimed loudly this time, tell her!

Even with this man's darker complexion, you could see his face redden then flush as tears began to form in his eyes.

I could see that he wanted to come forward to clean his slate. At once, he looked his wife dead in her face and said, "When I was a child, I was molested by my aunt and my niece on several different occasions." Bam! In your face with that truth. You could have used a crane to pick up the jaws that hit the floor that day. Was I shocked, not in the least? His wife's mouth dropped open and her eyes became moist as mine.

She got up from her side of the table with a slight nudge from me and went to hug her husband. You see it was not that he was a lazy dad who believed that all women should do the diaper changing. Inside he was still battling the demons of that little boys hurt of stolen innocence. It did not matter that the perpetrators of this crime were male or female. What mattered is that something great had been removed from his heart and he didn't even know how in a loving relationship how to recover it.

It was not the fantasy of grown men envisioning sex with grown women. It was not the excuse of a Radical Feminist society of, "maybe he enjoyed it." What he believed was that if he touched his own infant daughters naked body, that was attached to the same body that had been molested then maybe he would molest.

The Frankenstein Monster that had been planted deep within his damaged spirit to molest could possibly come out he thought. Truly this is not the case for all children that have been molested but it is the reality for many. The reason why I write this book is that instead of healing on the adult male side of life, maybe we can get into some prevention up front on these realities.

If there is one thing, I have found out in over two decades of teaching this course is that if you do not love someone where you found them, in the condition you find them they will never trust you. Just as in this case when the husband revealed that little secret to me in the presence of his wife but not in the privacy of their sacred marriage. In his behaviors of keeping what he considered a forbidden relationship secret indicates he did not think that she had the compassion to understand and deal with such a wrong without fleeing his side. Remember, they had been married for over nine-years and dated much earlier than that. If you can't tell someone for nine-plus years in a row then why do you believe an infant, toddler or young child to broach this hurtful subject with you, the parent?

Why Don't Scientist and Feminist Attribute Bi-Polar Disease to Men?

There is nothing stranger in the world than seeing a man being brought up on charges or dismissed from a job for inappropriate behaviors with his female co-worker. Especially when you see that they were both engaged into a work-related tryst. I am not talking about one of the, "Me Too" incidents but one in which the female initiated the encounter she is now lodging a complaint against. Since as far back as I can remember women have always been just as nasty mouthed or touchy-feely as men on the job. Even as early as my days in the U.S. military I can remember female soldiers' mouths uttering saltier comments than any male I have ever known.

The first thing you look to do as a male is to remove yourself from the situation as all men believe that women enjoy the protections that men are penalized for. These women know they can say and do as they please and there is not a damned thing that we can do about it. It is her word, against ours and in an equal world that means she wins. I can recount for you at least twelve times on the job of being touched inappropriately by women and this is just in my military career. I won't name for you how many times I could meet the standard of what feminist call sexual harassment outside of that.

The one secret that all of the females know full well is that nobody would believe a male over a female perpetrator. They knew that even if a superior officer caught them in the act, all they had to do was act immature or maybe cry to get out of being admonished. I faced the same practices by women on my civilian jobs so much that I no longer believe in a one-sided sexual harassment policy. Unlike other men these days, I have the luxury to work for myself and not to deal with that form of leadership or coworker.

For the longest when a man either files a complaint or report of sexual inappropriateness, it is either laughed off or dismissed as something he enjoyed.

Once again, I say to you that the modern-day feminist has stolen the play book of this country's most segregationist racist person from the past and applied it to her behaviors. She feels she should not be touched for the same things she finds offensive. Does this sound like behavior from the Old South? She blames her misdeeds on the victim and not herself. Sound like the Old South to me.

She believes that her counterpart should be brought to trial while she has immunity by virtue of her gender; a racist in the past would have used his color. What does equal mean when you can hide behind the difference that you say makes you the same? In modern, post-feminist world women still, use sexuality on the job to profit or off to steal from men. One would ask, what do I mean by saying that feminist use sex to steal or profit from men, but they do? I ask you; wouldn't this be an equal time in history where such things did not matter with income and privilege being equally available to both?

This would be true if the modern-day feminist didn't want everything that was hers and what her male counterpart owned at the same time. Let's look at some of the examples of any modern-day woman who purports to call herself a feminist using sex as a means to financial privilege. When you see me refer to the characters of feminist or radical feminist, I don't mean a particular set of women but all women.

As I said in chapter one, that a man out of his shortcomings chooses a woman based upon her body, looks or ass. But a woman out of her shortcomings picks a man based upon his power or income. So, let us take a look at the dating Radical Feminist and how money plays into her choice for men. Sure enough, when a working woman meets a perspective mate, she may have no clue as to what his income is but she has a general idea. The average female is in the place of potential male suitors because she has been taught the skill of accidentally placing yourself in front of the man you desire. In essence, she has to work hard at making the initial meet look like his idea instead of hers. She wants the man she pursues to think, "I am in this bar because I love warmed over beer and bad sports in a smoke-filled room." Females have been encouraged since before the dawn of liberation to get out and place her web where her potential male prey of high income frequents.

This means if you want a doctor, you should find the place where doctors hang out. If you want a politician then you need to find the places where they frequent. In this first instance, it is not as much as climbing any form of social ladder but jumping directly to the top of it. By now, I am sure you are saying that women are in the position to where they can become doctors themselves and they don't need to chase doctors.

This is just as true as a wife works and a husband should be able to go home for the rest of his life while she climbs the corporate ladder instead of him. Not! Most marriages and dating situations are predicated on the man having money as power and the woman having sex as power; still today. "You've come a long way baby," but I think you missed the last exit.

When a woman who is taught by novels, romance movies and every magazine at the checkout counter about males she sells herself short. Men are none of those things that are printed in articles for women genre. But if you are a guy, I want you to know that the woman you now live with or are currently dating your meeting was no accident. In most every crafted sketch of a romantic scene has a damsel falling into the arms of the beau she desires accidentally. When she can't get his attention, she is encouraged to place herself in front of him or bump into him accidentally.

Women know the one thing that guys do not, and that is that when we are about our life, we are not thinking of them. If we are not thinking about them, they can pass by us totally naked and we wouldn't notice them. So, it is this tired old stagehand bumping routine that has accompanied the birth of love throughout history and tomorrow morning. If you are a guy and are reading this portion you can look back over your lifetime and see how many women accidentally bumped into you. Now every occurrence is not this purposeful but who can tell with this type of scheme.

The bar room scene is now set. You have frequented this watering hole many times and she has put her feelers out to find out what type of person you are, where you work at and how much you make. You get up to go to the bathroom and before you know it bang…I'm sorry, I got to be more careful.

You lock eyes with her and apologize for bumping into her. In an instant, you believe that you have found the one beautiful girl that was missing from your life. She sweeps her hand through her long flowing hair, and they cut to the credits with the song, "Love lift us up where we belong, form the movie, An Officer and A Gentlemen." Maybe not, but you'll get the message.

All rights reserved, Paramount Pictures 1982

Most of these quickie love scenes end up with the Radical Feminist arguing with you each and every day you're together. She quite frankly does not know how to proceed with the relationship after setting it up because those movies and novels don't go that far. The only thing you can get from any one of those fantasies is make-believe happily ever after…roll to credits.

Her biggest awakening will come within two weeks once she wakes up beside you and realizes that she hates all men and especially you. She hates all men because she has been groomed to do so by her mom, the television, her friends and all those other devices I named for you previously. She believes that you were the one that had the Suffragists arrested and locked up in D.C. arrested on November 10, 1917, for picketing outside the White House for the right to vote. Although this is completely impossible as you are her exact same age. She mistakes the power of men in leadership positions for the power of men on the average street level.

Although you are her exact young age you also had the inside track at the Supreme Court of the United States a hundred years ago to uphold such nonsense. Yes, you are the one to blame. The boy who has always supported his single mother and in no way has ever disrespected any women. In fact, you don't agree with everything that went on back then or now. If anyone between both of you is approaching this moment in the wrong way it is, she.

For she was the one that shadowed you down a couple of weeks back in a dark smoky bar. It was she that had the intent to marry you, give you two children in a suburb home surrounded by a picket fence. This tired and most antiquated fantasy taught to all little girls is the basis of a split personality when it comes to women upholding feminism.

But the insanity doesn't begin to end there. Now that she thinks on it a moment maybe she was fooled into this entire relationship, and maybe by you. Hell, you aren't even her type. Why you don't look anything like the air-blown male models that are drawn on the front of those fictitious romance novels. You are long from ever having the pecks or flowing locks of Mr. Fabio Lanzoni.

She had better get out of this relationship as fast as she can before someone gets hurt. Only if she knew that it was too late for that the moment, she framed this love scene. What she has no clue of is unlike those pretend romance novels you are a living breathing human being. Males for the most part in my estimation are ready to, as they say; settle-down earlier than their female counterpart. I know that is a hard thing for women to swallow, but believe me, this is true.

If an adult male invite you into his home past a one night stand it is not always about sex. He does not need you to get sex in a world where anyone will have sex with you to include his same gender. In a world filled with phone pornography, prostitutes, call-girls and don't forget his left and right palm on a cold winter's night. No, when a male lets you into his world, if you don't ruin the invitation means he is probably serious. In my experience, I have watched young boys who grow into men flip from a public-school behavior to an adult like one. Females in school are more serious about some of their immature relationships where the human male is not.

Boys are into whoever has a hole on their body in school and is a willing participant to sex. Now after high school graduation and the seriousness of life hits both genders their stance against the opposite gender's switches. Most young adult males will be more into a relationship over merely a one-night stand. I bet you no romance novel or cheap magazine at the check-out stand will tell you that. When boys are dating in high school, they don't see themselves as spending their hard-earned income or time on a girl. But let that same boy move from an adult dating to married situation and watch what he will do with that same time and income. As a man, he will bring home even in the modern day his entire income for his family before he places himself first.

The only thing wrong with this is that most young adult men choose exactly the promiscuous young women they would have in school. Somehow after all we have witnessed concerning wives acting like children on their husband's time, we still believe that women mature before men. Actually, science has proven, time and time again that females' mature body wise before their male counterparts but the jury is still out on meeting your mate in the middle where responsibility lies. I can't tell you how many times I have seen young men with the best intentions choose young women with the worst intentions for them.

I can remember a young man who had everything going for him for a guy his age. But his choices in women were juvenile. The young woman he invited into his life ruined it although they were age matched. He gave her the keys to his house, access to his bank account and car. After the grace period in which females feel they have to fool men that they love them passed she let her real self-loose. She argued with him by phone every day when he was at work and finished up the pointless discussion after he arrived home.

When he was at work in order to get revenge for her perceived slight, she took his priceless collection of glass turtles and threw them through his priceless glass table. She then damaged his car and took off into the night without telling him where she was going. I thought for sure that he would have left her alone and glue his life back together. I believed he had learned his lesson and not to choose a woman in the future with similar traits, but boy was I wrong. Three months later he had that young foolish woman back in his home for round two. Long story painfully short, she broke his remaining collection on the way out. In fact, she took one of those priceless turtles and through it through both windows of his patio. She began to throw each one of them on the back lawn which abutted neighbor's back yards.

Since he was not home people started helping themselves to his priceless collections. The scariest thing about the whole affair was that this was in an upscale community. She cleaned his entire bank account out and took off. His landlord who was tired of the whole show immediately evicted him upon his arrival home that afternoon.

So, you see today I can't side with the feminist view that it is more in a man's best interest to get married than a woman. Males have plenty to lose by getting married. They can lose their home, their car, their job and everything they held dear before they decided on love. As the reader, I am sure you know or have one of these nightmarish stories concerning the couplings of the two genders.

Additionally, when a guy allows a woman to move into his apartment or home it is implied that she will not be paying for much of anything. How is this equal again? The woman that pays nothing on a guy's time is just given another chance to save for herself, retail therapy herself or take care of one of her friends on his time. If that same female had moved in with her girlfriend of the same age, she would be expected to pay half of the rent, the electric, cable and the like.

She would not be expected to feign helping with her income and then when the male does not insist ever help again. In any other form of civility, this would be called a bum, not a lady, not a girlfriend or a wife. Anywhere else in life they would throw you out on your ass just as they would a male. But in this current governmental environment, women are even protected in their wrongness.

Now for the young adult women and their choices after high school. A young adult female without the benefit of seasoning towards humanity is the last person you would want to move into your house, date or marry as a young man. I have spent the better part of three decades in a career that I tried in earnest to keep couples together.

As of today, I can tell you that I cannot and will not encourage a young man today to get married. Should he choose a young woman his age he is choosing a woman who is ready to have sex and experiment with more people than him. She feels that she has missed out on her high school quota achieved by her slutty girlfriend with boys.

In her opinion, all males cheat around and are dogs. They are people not to be trusted despite she is doing everything she projects onto them. Once she is in a relationship, she finds herself quickly out. If it is not her attitude it will be her desire to have sex with as many different men as possible. She reads her new man the riot act that women too should be allowed to play the field while being in committed relationships.

What she does not know is that if she should slip and get one disease from the many men that she refers to she could be maternally sterilized for life. She could pass on a disease to her unborn child further down the road. Playing her version of the male game could get her a sexually transmitted disease that could potentially end her life and the lives of everyone she slept with. Does this make her a bad person, no, just a mass murderer?

Young adult females in a relationship don't trust their young male counterparts one bit. They try to train them to childlike honesty while they do adulterated dishonesty. If you are a mother at this point with a grown man you know what I mean. Mothers with boys have a different phone call than mothers with daughters. A phone call from an adult son goes a little bit something like this. Hi mom, I know you told me not to get with her but she wrecked the car again. She slept with one of the guys at work and I got fired after we got into it. I don't know where she is now, but I am watching the kids. Can you come over and watch them while I go try to bring her home from her girlfriend's bar?

Whatever age you find the Blue Feminist in you will find a closeted hunger for sexuality. She would not have to keep the same desires she shames a male from if she would just be honest with herself. But she can't because all little girls are raised by women who tell them that they will be whores if they let their sexuality out of the closet. What they regret to tell them is these are all of the women that sleep with strange men at night just for the thrill of it. These are the same women that by daylight would swear that they are decent and men are filthy. Why do women primarily sneak around in the shadows in search of strange men not sanctioned by the government?

Women do this because they are on a cycle of sexuality hidden even from them. Unlike men, women's bodies have less than five percent testosterone during the day at any given time. Her testosterone levels peak during the midnight hour and then wean towards the early hours of the morning. It is during this midnight hour that most clubs see an increase of women wanting to have fun with the men they despise or would otherwise be repugnant by morning. I think most children that are born to mothers that they don't particularly like come from this midnight cycle of the fascination with strange men. Many years after the suitor has left the mother is left with the memory of someone that she can't stand.

Some women get pregnant accidentally because they are enjoying the risk of sex. Like the male, it is a kinkier risk to play with the fire of getting pregnant over actually getting pregnant. This woman will toss to the side those many governmental school classes about getting pregnant. Tonight, none of the Planned Parenthood pamphlets will fade from memory. Those birth control pills would just kill the risk of getting pregnant. The only thing that she will have to fall back on is a governmentally sanctioned abortion in about four weeks after her first missed period. By then all of the risk and kink would have gone right out of the window. Fear and self-loathing will rule the day her hormones ever thought that this was a thrill.

With the average cost of a first-trimester abortion running between $350 to $950 and a second-trimester abortion between $1200-$2100 and more and the third and final trimester in excess of $5,000 she finds herself in real trouble for a one-night stand.

To treat her for Herpes for one month can run anywhere between $14.00 dollars to $351.00 on sale.

To treat the outcomes of that same single night aids contact would be $855.00 to $3,535.00 dollars per month. Both of the prices are cost prohibitive to the man or woman who is barely getting by. The cost adds up if you combine a pregnancy with both STD's and complications. Luckily with the aid of the government, all but the abortion can be covered. I don't take these facts lightly, a joke or a jab at the mother. In my classes, I tell people that sex is the only sport that two go into a room together and come out with three persons. To this, I tell them to make sure you have your gear before you play the game if not; somebody is going to be injured and need hospitalization.

Once again, a governmental system of equality that seeks to fast-track women down a path of poverty and shame do not fix a problem, it causes a greater one. In a government-sanctioned competition with men women are trapped in the same addiction of online porn topped off with ordering discreet items to their house so no one can figure out their double-life. The very juvenile training given young girls when dealing with their male counterparts leads to confusion between both. The Blue Feminist will bait the average man on the job into a compromising position sexually only to turn him into management if he does not play her game. Operating in that same governmental protection system accorded to one gender over another he has no recourse beyond finding another job.

If she chooses to make life even more miserable for him, she can alert his new place of employment about the incident she staged. I know full well that women are just as nasty as men so I can't give credit to either, nor can I give protection to just one. On just about every job I ever had that mixed both genders; I have been touched, spoken to or dealt with sexually. I can't count how many times I have witnessed other guys I know being sexually harassed as well. But when it is a woman to man it is not considered sexual harassment. It may be considered a convoluted understanding of protective government regulation but not harassment.

One day we will decide for ourselves as a nation that equal really means equal. That the level-playing-field that every politician and feminist profess as a religion will become real for both genders. Without this protection accorded to both, we have little more than a similar weak oversite of the protections of the black man and woman during a Jim Crowe period of 1877 to 1955's Segregation. Only this time it is not the last century of idiocy we are talking about but men's rights in the year 2019.

I'm telling you that we are in deep trouble just as long as we try to regulate love as equal between the sexes. The chief reason that you can't legislate equality between the two is that every baby boy and girl is born blankly minded. They have no clue of a Constitutional Amendment or the hang-ups of a previous generation who are trying to find identity in something they will discover in your bedroom while you are in a conference meeting at work But our problems don't reside in the minds of children for I tell you that this problem has been baked into the minds of women.

When wives exchange natural sex with their husband for monies or control. When a woman tries to climb the corporate ladder by using her body suggestively or sexually. When an employer takes her up on that suggestion and she sues the company into insolvency. When a congresswoman uses her preferred national facial features over her male counterpart to get on the nightly news every day of the week.

When an intern uses her body to have sex with a cigar in front of a president. When a woman wants the law to protect her because she is a woman. Get a job because she is a woman, get an advantage anywhere over a male just because she is a woman. Yes, she can use sex in and outside of her bed without the support of the big government. But let's see what kind of damage big government in conjunction with the traveling sex sales-lady has done over the last forty-five years to destroy the definition of a man.

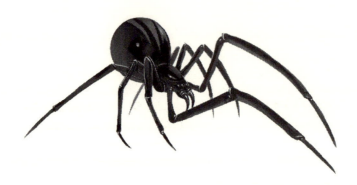

Black Widow Feminist
(The Toxic Mate)

"The Black Widow Feminist hides behind her gender after committing violence against her man. She can go from an aggressive posture to a victim in the time it takes the police car to arrive."

Charles Rivers

By now you must know that this book exists to reveal not only how Radical Feminist have altered the landscape of human relationships across the globe; but also that women are bad news. They are just as bad as they claim we are at hurting the ones they love behind closed doors. It matters not to me that women verbalize their ilk onto men or throw plates at their men who have no intention at hitting them back. Violence is violence and it doesn't matter in which form. In this chapter, I am going to be speaking out to the fact that mean women whether liberated or not can be cruel-hearted to their husband. For the longest time women have been ever so crafty to admonish their husbands behind closed doors as if they were his mother and outside of the home, make Jell-O molds for the school play featuring dancing trees.

I don't care how many governmental statistics you can quote me on domestic violence because governmental statistics alone don't truly paint a fair picture of anything. One of the unwritten codes that men have amongst one another is not to complain when their wives or girlfriends fuss and physically fight with them in private.

Today's woman is truly the perfect killing machine as in she can injure you and camouflage herself back into a sweet innocent make-up wearing princess. They use their demured stature when the police come knocking at your door or when the court system orders you out of your house. She uses that face and gender when she seeks to get a restraining order for the violence she has initiated with you.

By the time the average young female leaves home she has been conditioned by the same society that you grew up in that women are held in higher reverence than men. Women know this and proceed to beat the holy-shit out of their husbands or significant other behind closed doors. The behavior of the Black Widow Feminist is no different from the list of atrocities she equates to a violent male. There are times in the Black Widow Feminist month in which she is OK to be tiptoed around at her den. Then there are days when she takes out all of her work concerns and pains from childhood on her husband first and her children second.

The morbid thing about this entire deal is that society tolerates this type of behavior. Society as a whole makes excuses for feminine aggression while answering masculine aggression with a pair of handcuffs. In fact, we as a society have been taught that maybe her moods can be attributed to her monthly period cycle or her emotions. If you believe this to be true, then let me encourage you to throw out this line of reasoning for a new one. Let me tell you how I educationally arm men against the Black Widow Feminist when it comes to allowing this joke upon society to go on one more day.

You see I have found in counseling women that you have to be twenty steps ahead of her ability to lie to you. If not you will be lost in a whirlwind of excuses and lies. The first reason I don't tolerate home aggression or arguments in women is that a man's excuse for the same instance sounds ridiculous. Let us go back for a minute to the radical feminist main argument about domestic violence. I submit for you the drunk and abusive husband/father.

He has been made the poster child for every domestic violence law. Supposedly, he gets drunk, beats up on his family and then apologizes for it the next morning. He profusely promises that he will never do it again and ask for forgiveness. It was in this world that women were told to flee. It was from this world that women were told not to tolerate this type of behavior.

It was his criminalizing words of, "I only beat you this way when I get drunk." What about, "I only beat you this way when you make me mad." These statements are the first excuse I refuse to lend to women on their supposed time of the month or the up and downward swings of feminine emotions. For if I did allow women to get away with this, I would have to apologize to the drunk/abusive husband.

The second reason I do not give license to women's excuses for monthly periods any more than I do the drunk/abusive husband is that it can be controlled. The drunk father does not go to work drunk. He does not push around or beat up his fellow coworkers. He does not hurt them or apologizes in a lame excuse of, "the alcohol made me do it, or the devil made me do it."

Similarly, the wife who abuses her husband does not yell at her coworkers under the influence of alcohol. She does not kick her boss in the balls in a heated argument because she is on her period. She does not scream at her project manager because her emotions are going up or down. You see the female of the human species has learned since the beginning of recorded history how to make us look bad by making themselves look extremely good.

In doing this behavior no one ever expects that she is pouring hot water on you in your sleep. No one would imagine that she tried to stab you in a heated argument around the water cooler. And certainly, nobody at church last Sunday knew she slapped you for commenting back at an insult, she gave you. So, yes, Miss Butterfly who believes in saving the whales.

Miss. Caring, who believes in protecting women from domestic violence could very well start right there in her own damn home. It is high time to report these women who do this before they hurt someone for real and have you still being charged for domestic violence. Remember, she does not do this at the office or any place that the public could see her.

In fact, she is the most loved person in the office she works. She ensures that she lowers the respect level for her husband in the face of fellow workers. She does this so that she is not charged once they get wind of her true nature. Finally, they have Midol, Motrin, Pamprin, Tylenol, Nurofen, Premsyn, Advil and an endless amount of over the counter drugs for those type of mood swings. In short, if you don't do it at work, don't do it at home. Men are not the only homegrown abusers and its high-time that we start to bring this sort of violence out of the closet and into the main street.

As Men, we share an outdated unwritten pact not to admit that our wives are beating on us or throwing dishes at our heads in our private home. We have an unwritten code not to say, my mother, teacher, aunt, etc is molesting me. Amongst women, the vocalization of any one of these issues would be praised as strong in admitting what is happening in secret.

The same society laughs off, brushes off or pretends not to see what is obviously going on. Spousal abuse to husbands from wives has been going on long before women's liberation ever began. I ask, no, I beg you to use the same tactics of the feminist in these cases. Document your injuries and house damage with that smartphone you have. Call the police just as soon as she goes postal on you and has her evicted as she would you.

When you tolerate these behaviors from a woman that claims to love you she becomes intolerable. In truth, it is an accepted norm that maybe a man deserved it or he had it coming to him. As usual, I present for you one local story within the United States to prove that strength does not always rule the day when it comes to domestic violence. It seems to me that men's lives are expendable and their deaths, something to be glamorized when a wife kills her husband.

South Carolina woman killed husband by putting eye drops in his drinking water

By KARMA ALLEN Sep 3, 2018, 3:41 AM ET

A South Carolina woman was charged with murder after she allegedly poisoned her husband by putting eye drops in his drinking water, police said.

Lana Clayton, 52, confessed to killing her husband, Stephen Clayton, after an autopsy found poisonous levels of tetrahydrozoline in his system, the York County Sheriff's Office said Friday. Tetrahydrozoline is a chemical found in over-the-counter eye drops used to clear up eye redness.

Stephen Clayton, 64, was found dead in the couple's home in Clover, South Carolina, on July 21. His wife held a funeral for him in their backyard earlier this month before an autopsy uncovered his cause of death, neighbors said.

She later confessed to poisoning him, authorities said, telling investigators that she placed eye drops in his drinking water for several days. Lana Clayton, 52, confessed to poisoning her husband in the couple's South Carolina home. "I believe she's the one who called it in. She found him unresponsive in the house," Trent Faris, public information officer for the York County Sheriff's Office, told ABC News. "We don't have a clear cut reason why she committed the crime that she did, or what kind of motive she may have had. But we're still kind of working on that."

Stephen Clayton's family released a statement to ABC News saying they were "shocked and mortified" by his death, and attempted to debunk rumors the killing was precipitated by infidelity.

"The family is shocked and mortified at the cause of Steven's death.

All of our family and friends know how much he loved his wife Lana and how devoted he was to her. We are all still trying to process this," the statement said. "However, any references in media reports to a 2010 Facebook post by his wife having to do with an infidelity issue was centered around an ex-husband, not Steven who hadn't even met her until 3 years after that particular Facebook post.

"The family is respectful of the ensuing judicial process and does not want to make any statements that might jeopardize the due process of this case and those involved," it added. Stephen Clayton was found dead in his home in Clover, South Carolina.

Residents in the quiet town of Clover, near the North Carolina border just southwest of Charlotte, said they were shocked by the man's death. One neighbor said Lana Clayton attended a neighborhood Bible study and Stephen was known for his big personality, according to Charlotte ABC affiliate WSOC.

"It just makes no sense," Deborah Pollard, who lives nearby, told WSOC on Sunday. "That's crazy. ... They're just finding all kinds of ways to do crazy things nowadays, aren't they?"

Lana Clayton was booked into the York County Detention Center on Friday on charges of murder and malicious tampering with a drug product or food, police said. Jail records did not indicate if she had obtained a lawyer as of Monday morning.

-Police have not released a motive in the case.-

As you can see in this previous story the myth of man as abuser based upon size does not exist. You can be as small as a tube of eyedrops to take out a man weighing almost two hundred pounds. We need to end the day in America where a slap or an argument from a wife is seen as a corrective tool for her husband and the same is seen as horrific when it comes from the husband. The only way I can expect to explain how horrid it is for a woman to treat her husband this way is by equating it to a mothers love for a wayward child.

True mother's in some instances are stuck with the unenviable job of raising a child that hates their guts.

A child that is either physically hitting on the mother or berating her every chance they get. Sure this woman knows that she can physically whip the child but she chooses not to out of love or fear of being an abusive mom. So what does this little shit of a child do once he knows what her boundaries are; but crosses them and her nerves on a daily basis. She hears from society and the media every day that, there is absolutely no reason that a mother should ever want to beat a child.

But every day she holds back from becoming a convert to the act of corporal punishment. A mother locked in such a tenuous relationship without improvement or relief can hardly wait until her child has attained the age of emancipation in order that she may set them free. This is the same speech that men are given by other men who consider abusing a wife who is of lesser strength. On the other hand, his wife is encouraged by her negative female friends to tell him, "I am not afraid of you, and I dare you to hit me!" All of this is what takes place in the blink of an eye in the worst arguments of your life with the woman who claimed in the presence of family and a government official to love you.

This one vilolence motivating sentence becomes a goat to the male's ego. His so-called mate at this moment is trying to get him arrested and removed from the home. Do women do this because they want their relationships to come to ruin, hardly? They do this because they have been subconsciously raised to hate the male gender over their entire youth just for being male.

It is beyond me today that most grown women encourage young girls in the ways of hatred under the guise of feminism. How they convince females that they are smarter than men. These divisive words and gestures do little more than help to make men feel that they are doing real, San Quentin prison time on the couch of their own living rooms.

When I think of the wrath of hatred that the Feminist Movement has brought down upon it my mind searches back to a classic space thriller.

I am drawn back to the movie, Star Trek II, The Wrath of Khans scene in which Captain Kirks nemesis, Khan is watching his son die within his own arms. Khan's son upon his death looks up at his father and says, "Yours is the superior intellect." I ask you, how can a modern woman profess to have a superior intellect or be smarter than a man; while carry on in the ways of a child?

How can a woman profess to be nicer than a man yet act crueler? Khans son in that moveie is questioning him even in death as to why they came to ruin if his intelligence was that much better than Captain Kirks. If I were that dying son facing a woman in that scene I would be saying, "Yours is the nicer more decent, loving gender."

I believe we are sitting on the tip of the iceberg when we can come out as men and tell what we have been tolerating in the closet called relationship. I have had the privilege of dealing with and listening to men as well as women my entire life. I believe I can speak for both now when I say we are done, and tired of the Slave Codes of 1667 and double-standards of 2019. The biggest weapon of the Radical Feminist is the ability to change their stance at a moments notice to defend a bad position. She thrives on the grey area of the law that protects the negativity of women towards innocent men.

Throughout this entire chapter, I am going to name many instances where the abusing feminist wife changes her stance to win an argument with her husband, the law, the courts and certainly the court of public opinion. Before I list a hundred slights that wives do to their husbands I wish to show you her double-sided nature as it appears on the streets of your town each day.

For you see from the clerk at your local ice-cream parlor to your female CEO treat their husbands with disdain while uplift most men and women outside of their homes. You can take the nicest nasal squeaking decent feminist you believe to know and watch her action at home with her family.

You would have no more idea than an elephant with hearing aids that this woman behaved this way. A woman will usually engage her husband in a regular arguments in which she lowers the octaves of her voice a few scales to where she sounds just as masculine as he.

She will run him down in nature and read him the riot act with peppered remarks that are sarcastic towards men. I'm sure at this point you are asking well what if he started the discourse? With that, I say you are trained to respond that way. Society is conditioned to defend the actions of the perceived weak immediately over the perceived strong. But I am not concerned, either way, I am concerned as to what she does once she goes out the door and to that career/job.

Women are the kings of the closeted abusers they paint men out to be. This same woman will go down to her job just after telling her mate to go to hell and wish everyone she meets on the way a pleasant good morning. Makeup and a natural pleasant demeanor to some extent allows women the perfect protective mask of the abuser. The mere appearance of decency she has allows her to do the worst things to him in anonimity. The attractive serial killer, Ted Bundy was allowed to blend into the crowd for the longest time without getting caught. Why? Because society at the time he committed his most inhuman attrocities was looking for an unattractive angry man with an axe to grind against women.

The feminist mate-abuser enjoys this same mask of anonimity or publicly perceived weakness to protect her from corrective eyes. Like a male abuser she tries to distance her husband from his mother and family because she knows one thing. She knows his mother is no fool and she can see that his choice of wife was a mistake. Mothers are different than sons in the fact that women don't fall for their daughter-in-laws based upon their asses or sexuality. The longer the abusive feminist can keep mom separate from son she can get away with whatever she chooses to demonically do to him.

Even if she gets caught in the act of physical or verbal violence she could blame it on her husband and play weakling. So the next time you visit your local coffee house and have a female barrista smile at you and give you the greeting of the day, wonder. When you next go to your local big box retailer and see the female manager, wonder. Wonder if on the end of that smile and; how may I help you" are you dealing with an abuser or manipulator?. If this girl is dating or married she is treating her man with far less respect than she is offering you in that simple cup of coffee. I would go further to say if you knew what type of person she really was you would not accept that coffee or anything else from her.

Double Standard Slave Codes for Men

In a live-in situation, dating or marriage these are the things that the average feminist wife does to a man but does not want done back to her. She would actually walk-out on her boyfriend/husband or call the police if he even showed the signs of breaking the Slave Codes in her presence. Most of the issues on this list women will justify as maybe he deserved it, but who deserves strife over love? Remember, these crimes are expectant commonplace for feminist wives. Even if the husband reports the incident to the police they won't get involved for something they would easily arrest him for. They arrest him for his perceived strength, but you don't need any vaunted strength to do the following.

1. A woman will open-handed slap her man without fearing retrobution.
2. She bleaches his clothing that she knows is important to him.
3. She keys his car knowing a paint job cost money.
4. She cuts his clothing up into small pieces.
5. She throws his clothing out of the window.
6. She walks out on him at the most vulnerable time of his life.
7. She robs his bank account of needed monies at a critical time.
8. She throws household items and weapons at him in an argument.
9. She breaks items around the house to show him just how angry she can get.

10. She witholds sex from him in an attempt to change his personality.
11. She turns his own children against him.
12. She saves money on the side to leave him before he has even done anything wrong.
13. She refuses to show him the same natural affection she gives away outside of the home.
14. She shows him no respect whatsoever.
15. She thinks doing anything for him is a bother or a chore.
16. She often tries to stay away from home to avoid him.
17. She keeps communication with old boyfriends.
18. She has emotional affairs with male strangers and male coworkers.
19. She fantasizes about being with other men while having sex with him.
20. She flirts with other men in his presence.
21. She complains incesantly even when things are going great.
22. She speaks ill-will against him.
23. She complains about always being sick, but only in his presence.
24. She tries to stay late at work so she does not have to come home to him.
25. She extends her retirement age so she does not have to retire to the same house as he.
26. She has moved to the room down the hall from her husband.
27. She places him on the couch to control him sexually.
28. She volunteers to agencies and groups outsid of thehome the love and peace she denies him.
29. She shows no interest in her own children.
30. She argues over the smallest things but overlooks the large damage she does to her own marriage.
31. She tries to get him to change perpetually to suit her needs while insisting she needs no improvement.
32. She sneaks purchases in the home in order to keep secrets from him.
33. She checks to see if he is keeping secrets from her like a detective.
34. She fakes oral sex with him in a dirty attempt to smell his penis for another woman.

35. She makes every attempt to go out with her girlfriend places she will never take him to.
36. She dances and flirts with men in the places she goes with her single girlfriend.
37. She takes drugs behind his back.
38. She masterbates to the same porno films she calls him dirty for behind his back and denies him sex as if she has a low labito.
39. She has the desires and actions of a single woman although she heavily convinced him to get married.
40. She makes him late for all of his necessary appointments.
41. She doesn't clean her own body except when she is either trying to impress another suitor or going to a doctors appointment.
42. She laughs off her every mistake but magnifies his as stupid.
43. She calls him the most vile names immaginable.
44. She acts like a spoiled child when dealing with him.
45. She takes care when using her car, but not when using his.
46. She won't let him touch what is called, "her stuff" but considers his items community property.
47. She damages his collectable or throws them out.
48. She won't buy him as much as a cup of coffee.
49. He couldn't hold in one hand the things that she has ever bought him but in contarst she needs a house to hold what he has given.
50. The last time she touched him with the caressing love of a woman was when they were dating.
51. She won't take his phone calls at work.
52. She won't take his phone calls when she is with her friends.
53. His phone habits are to be investigated but hers are a womans privelege.
54. The only time she dreses suggestively is when she goes to the club without him or to work each day.
55. She allows him to pay the rent without the assistance of her salary.
56. She allows him to pay lessser bills as well such as, the water, electric, gas and cable. In this way she can keep her monies fro shopping for new outfits to where to work to impress her friends.

57. If she spends her paycheck it will be on herself or her girlfriends.
58. She lends her friends monies sometimes without getting it back but charges him for the same courtesy.
59. If she gives him a gift it will be crappy or not at all.
60. She buys him ties and cologne at Christmas knowing that he uses neither and that she can return these items to enjoy the refund.
61. He can't trust her when she says she is not lying to him.
62. She lives a double life but sometimes follows him in her car to see where he is going.
63. She helps the neighbors in need with the needed resoursces from their shared home.
64. She bakes cakes and cookie for her office staff but never for him.
65. She visits her fellow employees in the hospital but won't visit him in the hospital.
66. She holds long grudges against him that she would let her friend go for doing the same.
67. She insist in getting even with him in hate but not in the issuance of love.
68. She pretends that she is doing him a favor just to be married to him.
69. He has two pair of shoes and she owns forty six pairs.
70. He has seven changes of clothing and she over two hundred.
71. He doesn't feel that she knows him or will ever try as much as the men she did prior to this serious coupling.
72. The only time he hears her laughing is with her friends.
73. She trust her friends and strangers more than him.
74. She takes all of her friends suggestions but filters his before dismissing them.
75. She gets mad when he doesn't take her advice.
76. She keeps very negative female friends behind his back and them separate from knowing one another.
77. She speaks in a hyper sexual manner with her friends but fakes a phony lady-like demeanor with him.
78. She tries to make him angry.
79. She tries to make him physically aggressive.
80. She tries to get him to fight with other males in a casual

public setting for no reason but to defend her bad honor.
81. She tries to bring him down when he is happy.
82. She abuses alcohol and says she is just trying to come down off of a bad day.
83. She takes off out of the house after making him mad until he calms down.
84. She has called the police on him at different times in their relationship.
85. She has had her brothers or strangers threaten him in oredr to control the way she manipulates him.
86. She pretends to be nice in public although she and he knows that she has a split personality.
87. She threatens him with and without weapons.
88. She argues with him in front of the children.
89. She justifies her behavior with a feminism line that this is what men did in the past.
90. She prevents him from watching what he wants on tv.
91. She won't allow him to watch what he wants to on TV outside of shows that are eith romantic or include scenes of women being murdered.
92. She reads sexualized or romantic novels incessantly but will never act these things out in her own home.
93. She cheers on in other men what she overlooks in his behavior.
94. She considers the strength of other men but gets mad if other women acknowlege his.
95. She gets angry when other women compliment him.
96. The only time she shows interest in him is if another woman desires him.
97. She never cooks for him but enjoys him cooking for her.
98. She has never helped to clean the house but goes next door to help the neighbor clean theirs.
99. She meets her friends for coffee and food without inviting him along or bringing him as much as leftovers back.
100. She comes in as late as she likes but clocks his absence if he is home one minute late

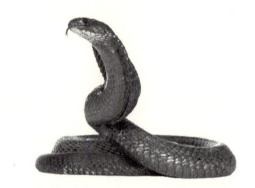

Cobra Feminist
(The Forked Tongue)

*"With her cold eyes and hypnotic sway,
the Cobra Feminist beckons the most gullible of men to join
her cause and help her defeat themselves."*

Charles Rivers

    We have been down a hate-filled road in this beautiful country many times before and it has only led to the death of innocent people and the destruction of innocent property. What we have failed to do even up till now is put a halt to the formation of these groups before they are able to do great mental damage. The radical feminist campaign has sought to stoke the fires of hate and discourse since the inception of its application to its local government.

Deceptive advertisers who had ignored female purchaser from previous generations in America decided to cash in on her newfound wealth through hate.

These companies were not stupid by any stretch of the imagination and wanted to enrich their pockets with her newly liberated income. A top tobacco manufacturer was applauded in the late 1900s when its top CEO professed, "We are only utilizing half of our audience." He was inferring that if society would only ease up on its morays about women smoking in public, they could have twice the number of customers. The big three manufacturers of tobacco began to trip all over themselves in their attempt to gain women as a new line of wealth.

Since they knew that the Suffragettes were fighting for women's rights, they decided to target that issue. They further proposed to focus their advertisement around the brewing hatred that women historically carried for men. From that day until now each and every manufacturer of women's products have cashed in on the gravy train of women are smarter and men are stupid. I challenge you tonight to watch the commercials on your TV with a little more than passive awareness. You will find that most companies that seek to sell a product to women have to profess that she is, **smart**. If the commercial has her play husband on it then it will insist that he is stupid. The advertiser is convinced that for someone to be smart the other person must be stupid.

Although there is absolutely no evidence to base this tag line on, one can hardly turn on entertainment without hearing this religion. Probably the number one up-hill battle I have to fight when picking modern day males' egos off of the ground is this belief of their inferiority to women. In truth, the main battle cry of the Women's Liberation Movement was a proposed trickery to alter the way boys think after they reach adulthood. In fact, the second top feminist in the movement decided to take a quote right out of the Bible and twist it. See her quote below.

We will raise our boys up as we shall have them to go and we will reap a new future out of that. We are tired of going to adult men for our rights. We will just create a crop of new grown men.

The Shrewd Feminist is a misguided woman who teaches women a falsity equivalent to what Adolf Hitler preached to German citizens concerning the superiority of ***The Master Race***. Notice that each time I bring to you a point about the feminist movement it matches a racial superiority design that is dangerous not simply for men but for the Caucasian male to which the Caucasian female originated from. It sounds like to me that this is a personal problem of infighting that a country is being used to propagate.

I want you to take a look at Adolph Hitler's definition of the master race that follows and you will see that it is the same snapshot that the Racist Radical Feminist campaign pushes with each year that goes by. In a minute I will tell you what I say to all men and women who tell me that women are superior to men. First off, I don't believe that any damn body is superior to anyone and I never have. There is but one way to find out who is superior if you can find me the person who can levitate above the ground instead of walk on it. Since all of us walk on the ground obviously we are all equal to one another.

The master race (German: Herrenrasse, also referred to as About this sound Herrenvolk "master people") is a concept in Nazi ideology in which the putative Nordic or Aryan races, predominant among Germans and other northern European peoples, are deemed the highest in racial hierarchy. Members of this alleged master race were referred to as Herrenmenschen ("master humans").

-WIKIPEDIA-

Hitler believed himself that one group was superior over another group until the Olympiad Jesse Owens demolished the myth of the Master Race in 1936 as Adolph Hitler sat in the audience. In that contest, Mr. Owens won a grand total of four gold medals and proved that no one is superior to anyone. The events he competed in were 100 meters, 200 meters, long jump, and 4 × 100-meter relays.

Ironically Jesse Owens at the time stated that Germans treated him better than Americans and Hitler better than Roosevelt. This is the damage that is to be expected in a country whose climate at the time was racism. Today we are presented once again with not an old racist attitude but a newer one under the guise of feminism.

There is no way to compare the genders with the difference in body chemistry and strength. It is as silly as comparing apples to oranges. What we need to be doing is making a coalition instead of a collision course with each other. But here is the true story I tell people who ask me about women being smarter than men. I know full well when these angry people approach me that they have their eyes wide open but the consciousness totally asleep. I ran into one such lady at a department store back in the late 1990s.

This woman carried a very terse dislike for her husband and the men of society as a whole. She came into the fancy department store I worked in as a shoe salesman in my youth. She let out insult upon insult about her husband and ending off by looking at me and saying, "but you know how stupid men are?" She did not mind a bit, to include me in on her misunderstanding of the roots of racism, sexism, and misandry.

At that moment, I could have chosen to go off on her if I was that type of person. But I didn't, although I wanted to. I stood there for a brief moment thinking about how my wife and children would have to eat mayonnaise sandwiches for dinner if I got fired by responding in kind to her attack. But here is what I said. I said, yes mam, I know exactly what you mean about men.

Men have at their own peril, cut down the forest in this country from coast to coast to build cities. They have designed and built every road in between and the inventions none of us can do without.

Finally, they made this very building we are standing in to include the air conditioner we are enjoying on this hot day. In fact, they designed the machinery that produced the clothing you are wearing today. Yes, mam, I know exactly what you mean about those stupid men. With this she walked away, unharmed but educated to the fact that everyone doesn't like sexism, no matter which gender is espousing it.

I have my entire life been against sexism on both sides of the chromosomes aisle but nothing irks me as much today as hurting innocent males in order to uplift females. You have little girls being raised to think that their male classmates are somehow stupid because they were born with a penis.

This is just as dumb as a former generation believing that girls were stupid because they were simply born with a vagina. The largest damage done is one day these young girls will grow up to be the bosses of the men they believe stupid. I ask you, how far you think a female boss would be willing to consider promoting a man that she feels is completely stupid. Probably about as much as the men who refused to hire women in the previous generation?

Boys today are made to believe that they are stupid because they do not know how many inventions have been made by people who were once their age. I have a game that I have developed for any feminist who believes women to be The Master Gender. The game is in two parts. You can play one of the games from your office or your home. The first game you must play outside. Anyone, male or female can participate in this game.

All you have to do is leave your house and go as far as the street curve to the sidewalk. You must place the palm of your hand down on that sidewalk to start. Now without raising your palm in a bent-over fashion begin to walk. You can lift your palm off of the sidewalk when you find something that a male has not built or invented. If it takes you going from one coast of the country to another your hand will be bleeding in short order. If you choose not to play the outside game you can play the inside game. The inside game is designed for the feminist or the woman who hates everything male.

I want you to go without for just twenty-four hours everything that a male has invented, designed or built in your day to day life. This means anything from your I-phone to the food you place in your mouth and everything in between. Doing this will serve a better response than marching down Pennsylvania Avenue in the city of Washington.

You see if anyone played this game, they would have to be hungry to starving, naked, thirsty, cold and susceptible to bugs biting them. They would be vulnerable to all sorts of attacks by strangers because you would not even have the police force or military. You would not even have the house you reside in now. There would be no faucet to get running water.

Forget about using that microwave because it would not have been invented any more than that stove you rarely use today or that refrigerator that has only left-over fast food. You could throw away those Tommy John stretch high-cut brief underwear and your toilet facilities to include Luvena fresh-wipes. The grass field that you would imagine yourself sitting in would actually be a forest with untamed animals running wild and running wild after you.

If you had survived natural childbirth you could only expect to live a short life span. Sure, there have been inventions of women throughout history but can we accept only those and do without the male inventors? If you say we cannot then why be we trying to undermine boys and men? Now, this is not sexism in the least because I have no respect for anyone that does not see women as total equals. I also do not have respect for anyone who tries to belittle males to uplift themselves.

Now I know there will be many people in America that will be wondering why I chose boys and men to motivate in this book rather than girls and women. My reason for doing so is because if I didn't, I believe I would go to my grave as a failure in life. Never before in the history of all of mankind, have little boys and men of all backgrounds been so vilified, marginalized, maligned, and yet so misunderstood.

The average male child beyond the age of infancy is seen as something that is a potential danger to his counterpart, "girl." But in making boys the national poster-child for re-training by governmental education has drawn a larger rift between the two sexes more than any one hate group ever could in the history of civilization. Because of this style of thinking parents have been encouraged to reeducate, medicate or at the very least be careful with young men in public. I don't know about you, but the last time such invasive rules were placed on one particular group over another it took a Presidential Proclamation to abolish these threats to liberty.

But we don't exactly need that to remedy this concern. For the problem of males not performing up to par cannot be lumped on governments or attacks on single mothers, any more than it can be on married couples that struggle to raise the next generation. Our problems rest in the loving of ourselves as Hitler preferred and the hating of others as the Klan and Malcolm-X preached.

Take for instance again the manufacturers smoking campaign to use women as an automatic slot machine of hate-filled dollars. Typically, the ad will be formulated around the hate you have for yourself or the hate you harbor for others. It is questionable whether smoking would have become as popular among women as it did if tobacco companies had not seized on this opportunity in the 1920s and 1930s to exploit ideas of liberation, power, and other important values for women to recruit them to the cigarette market.

In particular, they needed to develop new social images and meanings for female smoking to overcome the association with louche and libidinous behavior and morals. Smoking had to be repositioned as not only respectable but sociable, fashionable, stylish, and feminine. The goal was a potential doubling of the market. As described in 1928 by Mr. Hill, the president of American Tobacco, "It will be like opening a new gold mine right in our front yard".

-advertising slogan- **"She's gotta have it"** *-advertising slogan-*

One of the quickest ways to interest women in his product, Mr. Hill believed, was to zero in on women's waistlines. The timing could not have been better as slimness was coming into fashion along with bobbed hair and short skirts. The president of American Tobacco saw the potential of selling cigarettes to women as a fat-free way to satisfy hunger. The Lucky Strike campaign "Reach for Lucky instead of a sweet" of 1925 was one of the first media campaigns targeted at women (fig 2). The message was highly effective and increased Lucky Strike's market share by more than 200%. With the help of the father of public relations, Edward Bernays, American Tobacco made Lucky Strike the best-selling brand for two years.

-See the poster for this ad that follows-

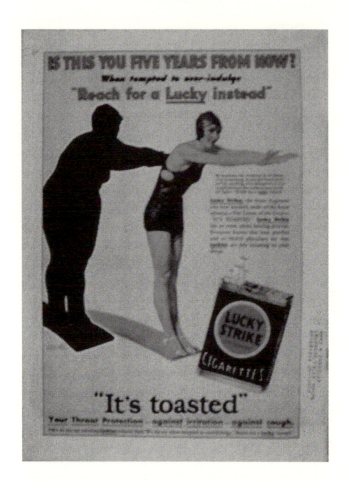

BMJ Journals website

Virginia Slims Cashes in on Women's Lib, Declaring: 'You've Come a Long Way, Baby'

Just as the feminist movement was gaining in strength and popularity, the Phillip Morris Company teamed up with the famed Leo Burnett Agency to capitalize on shifting attitudes. The campaign was for their new brand of ultra-smooth Virginia Slims cigarettes. It specifically and unabashedly targeted women, which was itself a new phenomenon. Every ad in the campaign put a woman front and center; equating smoking Virginia Slims with being independent, stylish, confident and liberated.

The slogan itself spoke directly about the progress women all over America were fighting for: "You've come a long way, baby." Women have indeed come a long way since the ads first crashed onto the scene, evolving past the surface traits of 1960s-era independence. "You've come a long way, baby" remains one of the most famous advertising campaign lines in U.S. history.

Article from A's website

One of the silliest births of hatred that helped contribute to women's advertising today is the Virginia Slims magazine advertisement. The ad featured after this paragraph seeks to sell an addictive cancer-causing product to women based upon their disdain for men. I have listed verbatim what the ad states so you can see the Feminist version of the movie, "Birth of a Nation."

"WE make Virginia Slims especially for women because they are biologically superior to men."

That's right, superior. Women are more resistant to starvation, fatigue, exposure, shock, and illness than men are. Women have two "X" chromosomes in their sex cells, while men have only one "X" chromosome...which some experts consider to be inferior chromosome.

They are also less inclined than men to congenital baldness, Albinism of the eyes, improperly developed sweat glands, color blindness of the red-green type, day blindness, defective hair follicles, defective iris, defective tooth enamel, double eyelashes, skin cysts, shortsightedness, night-blindness, nomadism, retinal detachment, and white occipital locks of hair.

In view of these and other facts, the makers of Virginia Slims feel it highly inappropriate that women continue to use the fat, stubby cigarettes designed for mere men.

-End of Advertisement-

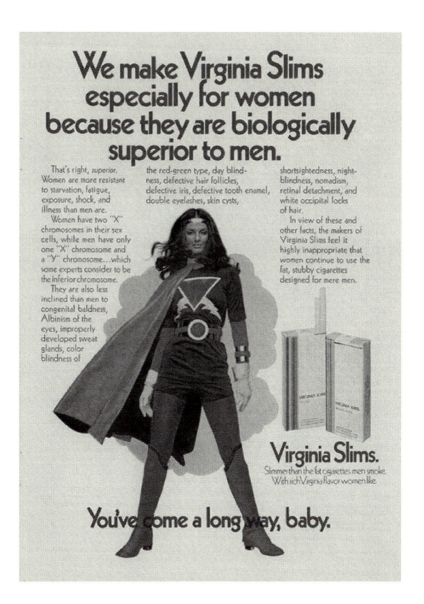

CHARLES RIVERS

ABOUT THE AUTHOR

Charles Rivers is a Southern California based Relationship Communication Specialist and Teacher. He is the author of, White Women Behaving Racistly, Lucid, Peace In Mind, Karma Shifts, Married without Baggage, The Good Marriage Maintenance Kit, How to Become Your Spouse's Best Friend, Apocalypse Angel and Heart of the Marriage. He has appeared on television in support of marital love and spoken weekly on a radio show entitled, "Relationship Thursdays." He is an army combat veteran and the winner of the Civilian Medal of Valor for bravery.

Manufactured by Amazon.ca
Bolton, ON